WINDOWS INTO TODAY'S
GROUP THERAPY

T0347107

WINDOWS INTO TODAY'S
GROUP THERAPY

The National Group Psychotherapy Institute of the Washington School of Psychiatry

Edited by

George Max Saiger, Sy Rubenfeld, Mary D. Dluhy

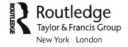

Routledge
Taylor & Francis Group
New York   London

Routledge
Taylor & Francis Group
711 Third Avenue,
New York, NY 10017

Routledge
Taylor & Francis Group
2 Park Square,
Milton Park, Abingdon,
Oxfordshire OX14 4RN

First issued in paperback 2014

Routledge is an imprint of the Taylor and Francis Group, an informa business

© 2008 by Taylor & Francis Group, LLC

ISBN 978-0-415-95843-1 (hbk)
ISBN 978-1-138-88169-3 (pbk)

Library of Congress Cataloging-in-Publication Data

National Group Psychotherapy Institute.
   Windows into today's group therapy / National Group Psychotherapy Institute of the Washington School of Psychiatry ; edited by George Saiger, Sy Rubenfeld, and Mary Dluhy.
      p. ; cm.
   Includes bibliographical references.
   ISBN 978-0-415-95843-1 (alk. paper)
   1. Group psychotherapy--Congresses. I. Saiger, George. II. Rubenfeld, Sy. III. Dluhy, Mary. IV. Washington School of Psychiatry. V. Title.
   [DNLM: 1. Psychotherapy, Group--Congresses. WM 430 N2774w 2007]

RC488.N37 2007
616.89'152--dc22   2007007156

Visit the Taylor & Francis Web site at
http://www.taylorandfrancis.com

and the Routledge Web site at
http://www.routledge.com

Dedication

Dedicated to the memory of our colleagues
Anne Alonso PhD
Hugh Mullen MD
Marvin Skolnik MD
whose extraordinary contributions to our field are only
hinted at by their essays in this volume.

Contents

EXISTENTIAL GROUP PSYCHOTHERAPY
Geoge Saiger

PSYCHOANALYTIC APPROACHES   171
George Saiger

SELF PSYCHOLOGY IN GROUP PSYCHOTHERAPY
Mary Dluhy

Acknowledgments

The editors and authors are grateful to the following for permission to reproduce their articles in this book:

Ramon Ganzarain. Introduction to object relations group therapy. *International Journal of Group Psychotherapy 42*(2), 1992. Reprinted with permission of Guilford Press.

Marcario Giraldo. Chaos and desire. *Group Analysis 34*(3): 349–362. Reproduced with permission from the author. © SAGE Publications, 2001, by permission of Sage Publications Ltd.

Irene N. H. Harwood. Toward optimum group placement from the perspective of the self or self experience. *Group 19*(3) 1995.

Earl Hopper. Group analysis and the study of maturity. *Group Analysis 33*(1): 29–34. Reproduced with permission from the author. © SAGE Publications, 2000, by permission of Sage Publications Ltd.

Molyn Leszcz (with Jan Malat). The interpersonal model of group psychotherapy. In *Praxis der Gruppenpsychotherapie* (ed. Tschuschke, V.). George Thieme Verlag, Stuttgart, 2001.

Malcolm Pines. The group-as-a-whole. In *The Psyche and the Social World* (eds. Brown, D. & Zinkin, L.). Jessica Kingsley, London. © Malcolm Pines 1994. Reproduced by permission of Jessica Kingsley Publishers.

George M. Saiger. Some thoughts on the existential lens in group psychotherapy. *Group 20*(2) 1996.

Michael J. Stiers. Containment and the threat of catastrophic change in psychotherapy groups. *Group 19*(3) 1995.

Introduction

This volume provides the reader with ways to think about group psychotherapy. It is a guide for both experienced clinician and novice, designed to facilitate critical thinking about theory. Though at different junctures it provides useful practical pointers and detailed clinical examples, its main focus is the ways different theories impact on the practice of the art.

It took some time before the importance of theory was recognized in the field. The pioneers—Joseph Pratt, Trigant Burrows, Louis Wender, and even Samuel Slavson—developed groups to meet pressing practical needs. Theory remained implicit. It was not long, however, before practitioners, often trained in the theories of psychoanalysis, began to articulate the underlying schemata of their methods. Early on, it became clear that it made an important difference whether a group was understood as a setting in which individual therapy could be accomplished or as itself an agent of change (or resistance).

In 1969 Morris Parloff, who wrote the epilogue to this volume, published an overview of the field, in which he described three major theoretical positions. He called these the "intrapersonal," where the focus remained on the individual and the goal was to effect changes in the intrapsychic structures and their internal balance; the "transactionalist," which focused on interpersonal relationships and "transactional" units; and the "integralist," where the major emphasis was on group process.*

In the decades that followed, the intellectual ferment that was part of the debate resulted in a fair amount of blending, of joining the best of each theory into a workable model. Few dynamic therapists worked without integrating

---

* Parloff, M. (1969). Analytic Group Psychotherapy. In J. Marmor (ed.), *Modern psychoanalysis* (pp. 492–531). New York: Basic Books.

individual, interpersonal, and group-as-a-whole threads into their practices. Intellectual excitement and debate remain alive and well, though. By the 1990s, theoretical innovation and refinement had led to the emergence of other schools of thought: systems theory, self-psychology, existential psychiatry, object relations, and Lacania psychology had joined a redefined group psychoanalysis and interpersonal therapy as leading ways of understanding the often-confusing welter of phenomena that took place within the unfolding of psychotherapy groups. This volume is dedicated to explicating and applying these theoretical approaches.

The Washington School of Psychiatry in Washington, D.C., has been on the leading edge of theoretical changes in psychotherapy in general. It has long offered a certificate program in group psychotherapy, The Group Psychotherapy Training Program, which had been founded in the mid-1960s. This program trained a generation of skilled group psychotherapists and formed a model for comprehensive group training. In the changing atmosphere of the early 1990s, the faculty became increasingly concerned that its program for teaching group therapy skills intensively to a select few needed to be rethought. The result, aided significantly by a grant from the Group Therapy Foundation, was the emergence, in 1994, of the National Group Psychotherapy Institute, which continues the tradition of challenging the frontiers of psychodynamic group psychotherapy. A new Institute cycle starts every 2 years.

The Institute emphasizes both experiential and didactic learning, though we could not capture the living, breathing quality of the former in this volume. We have included many of the important papers that it generated. These were delivered by both Washington School of Psychiatry faculty and visiting presenters. They well represent the various vertices from which modern group psychotherapy can be studied. Space does not allow reproduction of all the papers that were delivered, though at one point we thought this volume might be a record of the proceedings of the first three cycles of the Institute (1994–2000). Those we have chosen vary a good deal, as the reader will soon learn. Some are aimed at beginners in the field; others are highly technical. A few are already a bit dated, but their historical value alone led us to include them. We hope that we have made responsible and informative editorial choices in what we have included and omitted here.

The papers are organized according to theoretical position, as was each conference of the Institute. This has proven to be of significant heuristic value. However, the reader will become aware, as did the Institute members, that such divisions have inherent limitations. Reading the papers in each theoretical chapter makes abundantly clear that there is significant overlap and that theorists of one persuasion draw heavily on contributions made by others who define their views very differently.

No better introduction to this endeavor could be written than the paper delivered by David Hawkins, MD, which was delivered as part of an effort to integrate the various approaches represented in each conference, "Overview and Underpinnings." Each of the subsequent chapters will deal with one major theoretical approach, with one *vertex*, one way of viewing the enterprise.

Thus our title: *Windows Into Today's Group Psychotherapy.*

George Saiger

Overview and Underpinnings

David Hawkins

Introduction

Thank you, and hello. I am honored to be a part of this Third National Group Psychotherapy Institute. The conceptual depth and the academic caliber of this program make it an element that both sustains and advances the field of group psychotherapy. I congratulate you for participating in it.

Last weekend, I happened upon an exhibit of photographs and quotes taken from a dance therapy group for sexual abuse survivors. One quote in particular caught my attention. It read as follows:

> Out of my experience I would suggest two things. The first is to find some close people who will keep secrets and who you can share just a little bit with. By putting words to it you get the chance to get this terrible, blocked feeling out. Otherwise, it stays imprisoned inside you. And, I might add, manifests in all sorts of personal, interpersonal, and systemic symptoms.

I hope these heartfelt words will remind us of our goal: to learn how to conduct groups, using basic guiding concepts and user-friendly language, in which people can help each other improve their lives.

This topic seemed really exciting 2 years ago when I first accepted, but daunting when it came to putting the words together—not unlike the experience we all have when first trying to make sense of a group's process and respond to it in a way that hopefully will be constructive. How do we pay attention to manifest content, latent content, nonverbal behavior, and our own feelings? Can we imagine what Agazarian and Peters so aptly called "the Invisible Group," the roles being played in the service of developmental tasks? Then how do we integrate this data to determine whether an intervention from the leader is called for and, if so, what it might best be?

Whenever the thought of a group therapy T-shirt has come up, I have thought it should read "So many interventions, so little time."

I could tell you a bit about my own experience of integrating. I became interested in group therapy during my psychiatry residency. My group therapy mentor was an energetic, charismatic man who focused on techniques of working with individuals in a group setting. He returned from weekends with Albert Ellis or Cazriel full of excitement, sometimes startling his patients as he approached them from an unexpected angle or introduced new language and concepts to the therapy. I did see that he cared about his patients, they cared about each other, and, most importantly, they often improved significantly. I learned that there was hope.

I began to attend weekend workshops in transactional analysis and Gestalt therapy and then longer residential programs in these modalities. This training focused most on working with the individual in a group setting but also explicated interactions between people and looked at the family as a system. Two observations led me to think more about "the group." One was that there are many parts, or voices, inside each individual—a group, as it were. In this group, some parts might dominate or control, others defer or operate indirectly, and others stay so still and quiet that no one knows they are there. Somehow these parts had to work together efficiently for problems to be solved and symptoms to be relieved.

I also saw that, when they did, something rather magical happened: The whole group of parts became something more than it had been before. When they could join together and become cohesive, the whole really was greater than the sum of its parts.

At meetings of the American Group Psychotherapy Association I was exposed to other theories and styles of group leadership. I began to appreciate the concepts of the group-as-a-whole, the structural and cultural development of the group over time, and the group as a system.

These were exciting concepts. I could use them to better understand the process of the group and also the individuals in the group. As the group analysts say, "the group doesn't arise from individuals; rather, the individual arises from the group." Patients could use these concepts to better understand themselves and each other and to sustain their relationships through the inevitable difficulties that occur. They helped create understanding and integration of the deviant, discordant, unknown, or unacceptable parts and voices.

As I looked back on my journey, it seemed I had learned about group therapy in reverse. I decided that working from the vantage point of the group as a system first, and then moving to thinking of the individual in the group, was the most efficient direction for teaching and for constructing interventions.

Examples From My Work

I plan to cite some recent clinical examples, because they help bring theory to life. They come from several areas of my current practice. I see individual patients and work with three outpatient therapy groups that meet weekly. Six days each month I work with groups that utilize a different time format. These are therapy groups for mental health professionals. They also serve as experiential training in psychodynamic group psychotherapy. Each group of twelve meets for 6 hours, 1 day per month, and 10 months per year. Members usually stay in the groups between 2 and 7 years; some have stayed as long as 10.

I also lead consultation groups for group therapists in private practice and conduct group psychotherapy training for psychiatry residents from Duke and UNC. As part of this work, I supervise an outpatient group coled by two residents. I have followed this group for 8 years through numerous changes in its leadership. In addition to these clinical settings, my work in the governance of AGPA has been enormously challenging and instructive regarding the interface between the process of therapy groups and organizational dynamics.

An Integrative Approach to Understanding Time and Therapy

To move from these introductory remarks into a discussion of overview and underpinnings, I need to talk about the relationship of epigenetic development, change in group psychotherapy, and time.

Epigenetic development means that each developmental stage is built on the foundation of the more or less successful completion of previous stages. Many life events trigger our revisiting earlier stages. Thus, we travel through life in a sideways helix, reworking stages of development, hopefully completing some unfinished business within each loop and bringing more of ourselves forward in the process.

Change in Group Psychotherapy: Metaphor of the Hologram

1. Units of change happen in the moment, a fragment of the holographic plate.

2. Change is stabilized through repetition over time, adding fragments together for clarity.

3. Change of greater complexity is possible as a therapeutic culture matures; the culture is a frame, as it were, in which seemingly unrelated pieces of the hologram can be held until we are able to perceive the three-dimensionality of the subject of which they are a part.

I work primarily with semi-open-ended groups. In them I see the value of reworking the same material each time the group changes in composition and the value of prolonged periods of stability and sustained membership in allowing

the work to go to deeper levels. In addition, I see the value of developing a therapeutic culture that transcends many iterations of membership. This is especially
important when the group is working to metabolize cultural problems from the
larger society and to create change that later may be transported back across
the group's boundary and used to influence the norms of this larger culture. For
example, Virginia Goldner has reported on groups for couples in which a spouse
has been physically abusive. After a time, the group develops a culture that challenges dysfunctional gender stereotypes, which then changes the members' participation in perpetuating these stereotypes in the culture outside the group.

Constructing a Theory for Integration

Let us start with the premise that there are multiple ways to understand and lead
groups toward a therapeutic goal. However, in our development as therapists, at
some point we must choose one theoretical approach, learn it, and follow it. As
a friend of mine says, "If someone gives you a recipe, always follow it exactly
the first time." Having an open mind to consider information from different
approaches later is fine, but being "eclectic" to the point of losing, or never choosing, focus and orientation is not.

In this training program, you have heard about, and experienced, a number of
theoretical approaches. No one approach is "right." All have merit. Which theory and
style each of us gravitates toward depends, in part, on who each of us is as a person.

A second premise is that there are groups with different tasks, and therefore
different needs that might be understood best using different theories and met
most successfully using different leadership styles. Although it is true that "a
group is a group is a group" and that basic theoretical constructs translate from
one situation to another, we must also be aware that some settings call for special
techniques or training.

In the finishing phase of any training program, we face several important
tasks. We must appreciate the scope of our experience, assessing what we have
and have not learned. Although challenging and comparing are necessary for earlier stages of the learning process, finishing involves letting go of arguments used
to maintain a dependent position. The task at this point is to assume responsibility
for what we have learned and then put it to use.

The Process of Integrating: Maintaining the Therapeutic Environment

We take what we have learned, integrate it in some way, and go to work, "maintaining the therapeutic environment." To help ourselves through the difficulties
that we inevitably encounter, we need a set of basic concepts we can return to for
orientation and guidance.

The primary "basic" is *primum non nocere*. First, do not cause harm. In our
work as group therapists it is important that we understand how harm can occur,
develop skills to prevent it, and educate our groups about this process.

Yalom, Lieberman, and Miles gave us some very useful information in their book, *Encounter Groups: First Facts*. For one thing, they named the beast: group casualties, a particularly salient point in the era of encounter groups but no less a concern now. They pointed out that casualties were not related to theoretical orientation of the leaders but rather to certain leadership styles. The leaders with the least casualties paid attention to the following tasks:

- Maintaining executive function
- Encouraging interaction
- Providing meaning attribution

Executive Function

This basically means attending to the boundaries. It is the leader's job to be in charge of membership, the group's working environment, the time boundary, setting the working agreement, and monitoring the group's relationship to its task. This set of boundaries provides the frame that allows the group to focus on its task. Just as when we look through a microscope, the steadier we can keep the frame, the finer the detail we can discern within the field.

Encouraging Interaction

Jerome Frank wrote that a major component of healing was "restoring valued membership in a valued group." My goddaughter once told me she had written a book. Its content was "sometimes I play with Dawn and sometimes I play with Robbie," and other comments of that nature, all about her valued and valuing interactions. A patient whose fondest dream had been to have me interact with to her was the only member in group one evening. She spent the entire time talking about all the members she had come to know over the years.

The charismatic leader who is focused on being the agent of change may be most at risk for losing sight of the members' need to form, maintain, and value their relationships to each other, as well as their relationship to the group entity, which has often been referred to as "the mother group."

Providing Meaning Attribution

The third function involves meaning attribution. The antithesis of meaning attribution is the expression "This is just crazy." As Watzlavic, Weakland, and Fisch pointed out, problems are created by the way they are defined. To redefine them we must see them differently. It is very difficult to see what we cannot imagine. I think here again of Agazarian and Peters's *The Visible and Invisible Group*. It is our imagined map of the group as a system and of its structural development over time, as well as our capacity to conceptualize the group-as-a-whole entity, that most helps us create understanding around confusing and distressing individual, interpersonal, or systemic experiences.

The Map for Meaning Attribution

To create a map for meaning attribution, it is helpful to consider that there are four perspectives from which any group event can be simultaneously correctly understood:

- The individual
- The interpersonal
- The structural
- The group-as-a-whole

For instance, the common event of a member announcing that "this is my last meeting" could be understood as a repetitive pattern in that member's life, an interpersonal bid to be begged to stay or angrily told to leave, a challenge to the leader's authority, or an attempt to rescue a group that is teetering on the brink of intimacy.

So, if these perspectives are simultaneously correct, which do we use to construct an intervention at any given moment?

There is an old joke about the garage mechanic who charges $100 for hitting the engine with a hammer. He explains, "It's one dollar for the tap; ninety-nine for knowing where to do it."

Ezriel, who gave us the concept of "the common group tension," suggested withholding individual interpretation until the common tension was identified and then interpreting each member's relationship to that tension. Horwitz has suggested a modification in which the leader responds to individuals as the group session progresses and later discusses whole-group issues. I am suggesting, as an integrating principle, that whichever systemic level we choose to address, if we orient ourselves around the group as an evolving system, we are less likely to lodge a group issue in an individual or subgroup.

For instance, a new group member was complaining that she was unsure if the group could help her, which they tried to do, to no avail. Only when I pointed out (for the third time) that she was not the only anxious person in "this new group" could we join in the common tension that was being both experienced and defended against.

Throughout any group's life, be it short or long, changes occurring around the boundaries (including moving from one developmental stage to another) perturb the group members. When the leader facilitates recognition of such events and management of the accompanying affect, cohesion can be restored and understanding can be created. This is wonderfully reflected in the Schermer/Klein paper, which is not just about termination but also about interruptions and all the other boundary perturbations around which both regression and the work of separation/individuation occur.

Let me tell you more about the group I have supervised for 8 years:

> It is co-led by two psychiatry residents, one, and sometimes both, rotating out each year. Membership has varied between four and seven. Two of the members have been in the group the entire time. All of the

members hold jobs and are fairly self-sufficient, but all have recurring significant difficulties with employers and other authority figures, stressful relationships with family members, and few other satisfying relationships. Early in the group's life there were a number of suicide attempts, hospitalizations, and explosive job terminations. In the past few years, however, what was formerly put into action has much more successfully been put into words. Each time there has been a change in leadership, a similar pattern has been evident in the group's process. For several weeks there is talk of violence toward others or self, expressed wishes to go into the hospital and get away from it all, or fantasies of terminating employment. This is followed by a mourning period in which members express shame that they are still here and no better than they have ever been (which is not true), whereas others (I believe they mean the leaders) have gotten better and moved on. Following this expression of grief they return to an active interest in each other's work and personal lives.

During these transition periods there are often references to the group's history and stories told about past leaders, sometimes by members who never met them. One such story is about the Scandinavian man who was away from the group a month longer than planned because his visa expired while he was visiting his family. I wonder if this story is important because he left them, the fault belongs to him and to an authority above him, and he did return.

One co-leader was a shy African American woman who, despite her reticence, was an excellent beginning group therapist. Though she was well liked by many group members, she is seldom mentioned in these historical reviews. I wonder if this is because she rotated out of the group late in her pregnancy, choosing to care for another baby instead of the group, and the affect around her loss is not easily approached. She was replaced by another African American woman who, unfortunately, was the only resident I ever had to ask to leave the group, which she did with relief. Her narcissistic defenses were so brittle that, as she painfully confessed, she could only see the group members as "a bunch of losers." This resident is remembered by the group, and I am sure she carries some negative transference from her predecessor. In fact, we must wonder how her attitude influenced the group's relationship to her while she was in the leadership role. I, of course, must wonder if I misunderstood material that might have enabled us to work this through sooner.

More recently, the group was co-led by a man from Taiwan and a Caucasian woman. Both seemed to connect well with the group and follow the material, but they each had trouble maintaining the beginning time boundary. Listening to process notes, I heard mounting agitation among the members. Then both therapists managed to miss the same group meeting. The members were quite resourceful, attempting to page both leaders and staying for most of the session. By the next week, however, the group was definitely in fight flight, splitting into subgroups and voicing threats of leaving in response to each other's behavior. Miss E began to feel more and more injured and misunderstood by any comment addressed to her, even positive ones. Mr. L and Miss K threatened, before Miss E arrived one evening, to leave if she acted that way one more time. In the ensuing session, Dr. A asked the group to give Miss E "feedback" on her inability to take a compliment. They readily jumped to the task.

This is an example of the danger of an intervention at the interpersonal level when one at the group-as-a-whole level is called for. Regrettably, it is not an unusual mistake. It illustrates a failure to maintain executive function—in this case, boundary maintenance—and to provide affect regulation by normalizing feelings. In addition, it shows how a potential group casualty can be caused, through the process of scapegoating, when the group is not facilitated in metabolizing an overwhelming experience.

In the supervisory session, I said that the problem was not that Miss E could not take a compliment but that the leaders were not being responsible for an important part of their job and could not take "the heat" for their mistake. At this point the leaders "got" what they had been missing and began to refer to their having abandoned their job of maintaining the group's boundaries. After several sessions, Mr. L, a sometimes-violent man who blames his father for not protecting him from sexual exploitation, exploded verbally: "I am sick and tired of you trying to take the blame for this group's troubles . . . I do not need a wimpy-assed therapist." Not surprisingly, the group calmed down and returned to expressing interest in each other's lives.

This example can also lead us to consider the container phenomenon and to wonder about the difference between scapegoat and protagonist. In a psychodrama group, sociogramatic exercises are used at the beginning of a session to "warm up" the group. During these, a kind of cohesion develops and the group is able, mostly unconsciously, to elect a protagonist whose work will somehow speak for all of the members. In a psychodynamic group, with each session or new developmental phase, the group must work to reestablish cohesion. If someone either is "elected" or "volunteers" to become the focus of the group before this is accomplished, they are likely to serve as the container of an issue. In this case they are not working for the group; they are working instead of the group, and consequently they are at risk. It is the leader's job to recognize symptoms of "container-ism," or individual overload, and to engage the rest of the group in assuming ownership of their portion of the issue. In a maturing group, or at least on a good day, the group will assume this function. Let us return to the group I was describing earlier.

The group has been informed that Dr. A will be leaving at the end of the academic year and that the male co-leader, Dr. C, will bring in another co-leader during the summer. At this point they are not discussing this openly, focusing instead on Miss E's trouble with her new boss and the potential loss of her job. Late in the session, Mr. L recounts, with growing agitation, a run-in with the African American manager of a fast-food restaurant. He seems to be directing his story to Miss E, who, perhaps fearing a return to the scapegoat role, suggests he might look at the empty chair next to her instead. Just as the group is ending, Mr. N refers to the chair and wonders when they might be getting a new member. Mr. L, by this point quite worked up, says, as he exits, "Well, if they bring someone Black in here, I'm not staying in this group."

The next session began on a subdued note. Mr. L asked Miss E about her job. She reported that she would, in fact, be terminated and that she had already applied for other open positions in the system where she works. This, by the way, is very new, quite self-reliant behavior for Miss E. Other members were supportive and soothing and did not agitate themselves by focusing on her boss, as they would have in times past. They did feel that Miss E was being treated unfairly, however, and entered into a discussion on the process of scapegoating, including its biblical derivation. They wondered how people became scapegoats, and Mr. N told a Japanese expression, "If a nail sticks up, hammer it down." He said this meant that difference would not be tolerated. The group then discussed how it was the responsibility of others to help out when they saw someone being scapegoated.

An interesting metaphoric shy occurred, and the group began to give examples of people being victimized in movies. Miss E, who feels very unattractive, expressed her hatred of Gwyneth Paltrow for being so thin. Dr. A, who looks a bit like this actress, noted that even a "good" quality could be scapegoated.

As the time to end approached, the members seemed calm, interested in each other and in the topic. Someone noted that a new member coming into a group that had been working together for a while, as they had, would probably feel "different." They concluded that it would be their job to help the new person feel more comfortable.

In this session it seemed that Miss E, no longer in the scapegoat role, was actually in the role of the group protagonist.

Other Integrating Concepts

There are certain things always going on in the life of a group, whether or not our theoretical orientation leads us to focus on them.

A group is part of a larger system, and therefore it embodies conflicts and issues that exist in that system. In my consultation groups, we always lead off by considering how long the group in question has been in its current configuration, what has happened developmentally, what we know about its culture over time, and what else is going on in the system of which it is a part. This system may be an agency, a training program, or someone's private practice. Very frequently, after we have clarified the problem, an additional "oh, by the way" piece of information about the system is brought forth.

> In the group we have followed through several examples, Dr. A's difficulty with starting the group on time was, as most such things are, multidetermined. There had been several mentions of schedules being disrupted by having to wait for supervising psychiatrists on the Consultation Service. Besides being a reference to our relationship, this indicated a systemic problem with honoring time commitments that had not been confronted. It was therefore being passed on to the group. It helped the residents to realize that this is a very common problem in such systems and that it is our job as group therapists to educate the system regarding the conditions necessary for responsibly using this modality and to support each other in this work. I also offered to talk with the other faculty, if need be, to help protect their time with the group.

The parallel between this example and the situation many clinicians face in the current mental health delivery system is pretty obvious. Many consultations reveal that feelings of disempowerment within an agency, or frustration at having made a "pact with the devil" with managed care, have caused the therapist to act out in relationship to the group.

Transference

Though transference and countertransference are not the major focus of my presentation, I do want to say something about the richness of transferential possibilities in group therapy.

Transference and projective identification occur in three different areas, or across three boundaries: toward the leader, toward other members, and toward the group-as-a-whole.

Transference Toward the Therapist

In Winnicott's terms, the group therapist must be available to be both object mother and environmental mother. At times we are in the patients' central vision—intensely hated, loved, feared, desired, or envied. At times we are in their peripheral vision, hardly noticed as the group proceeds or, worst, discarded like an old orange peel (his words).

Both positions stir interesting countertransference that we must be able to recognize and manage.

Transference Toward the Group-as-a-Whole
Work with transference to the group-as-a-whole depends on our capacity to imagine the group entity, facilitate group members' relationship to it, and honor its importance to them. This area of transference, in my consulting experience, is most often underside or misunderstood. Work in this area offers great potential for the development of object constancy.

Examples of Group-Related Dreams
- A woman whose mother had recently died had a dream in which the group was preparing a meal. She mentioned four members in particular, and the group noticed that these members' usual seats were "like points of the compass," providing orientation in a disorienting experience.
- Prior to a vacation break, a man reported he had dreamed he was talking to his mother. He said, "I know my mother is actually dead, but I was talking to her anyway." Exploration confirmed this as an expression of his developing object constancy in his relationship with the group, which would be there over the break even when it was not.

Learning to Be a Group Therapist

I would like to say a few things about learning to be a group therapist and maintaining a therapeutic environment in our practice. Gaining competence in this field is like learning about a neighborhood, walking around it until we can orient ourselves in the dark. In doing so, we are learning human life skills that become a part of our way of being. (I refer you to the lovely quote from the brochure, "Groups are fundamental etc.") We learn best if we can experience group life from several different vantage points: member, leader, coleader, observer, and supervisee. It is also important that we provide ourselves with continuing education, supervision, consultation, and opportunities to reexperience group membership. This is not really about learning "how to do it," in a linear fashion. It is about valuing the complexity of human interaction and honoring our need for help from others in creating meaning.

We contribute to maintenance of the therapeutic environment by participating in the community of group therapists. Affiliate society newsletters, for example, help remind members that "there is a there there."

We contribute by speaking for the modality.

- Educating patients, the public, and other professionals. For instance, a psychiatry resident mentioned in one of the examples used information from her group supervision to improve respect for time boundaries by others in her department.
- Standards and certification. Many patients and other professionals have little understanding about group training and credentialing. Our job includes obtaining adequate training ourselves and educating others about its necessity.

The Culture of Group Psychotherapy: A Transportable Commodity

The Culloden Group

Group psychotherapy works best and is used most readily in a system where it is understood and valued. Clinical service delivery systems, training institutions, and communities of therapists vary widely in this regard, from those where group treatment is hardly known and group referral is seldom considered to those with rich resources for referral and training. Among the former, it is not unusual to find group therapy regarded predominately as a procedure, one for which training in individual therapy is sufficient preparation. Among the latter, the process of group treatment is valued to the point that its important components are integrated into the lives of its practitioners and used not only in therapy but also in dealing with the many group situations in which we all must participate. Furthermore, this culture becomes an exportable commodity that can influence other systems. A lovely example of this is the work of The Culloden Group. This international effort was begun as a joint effort by group therapists from the Boston area, which has a highly developed psychodynamic group psychotherapy culture, and therapists in Belfast, Northern Ireland, where the experiential aspects of group therapy training are less well inculturated. The group's goal is to bring group psychotherapy training to Northern Ireland through an annual institute and conference and also to bring the values and potentially healing experiences this therapy contains to understand and perhaps influence a social system that has struggled with deep sociopolitical conflict. Because the psychodynamic culture contains the belief that the group teaches the leader, carrying a wisdom that the leader must learn to understand, this effort is structured not as the Americans helping the Irish but rather as a truly mutual experience. Having participated in this venture, I greatly value the windows of insight into individuals (including myself), cultures, and the working of group dynamics that it has provided.

> In a sociopolitical setting in which self-revelation was unusual and potentially dangerous, a large group of 50 conference participants from America and Northern Ireland, facilitated by two group analysts, struggled to express the tensions in the room. It was the first anniversary of the bombing at Omagh. This shattering tragedy had occurred on the last day of the conference the previous year. In the ensuing discourse many versions of "poor relation" were explored. Were the Irish the "poor relations" the Americans were coming to help? Were the American visitors who had reacted emotionally to the bombing the "poor relations," unentitled to their feelings because this was not, after all, their tragedy? Were the "poor relations" those Irish who had left to create new lives in America, or those who remained? And, of course, could the "poor relations" among the many subgroups in the room be brought to a sense of repair?

There was little way to be present without strongly experiencing the many painful sides of life contained in this group. Although such a complex event could not be expected to end with resolution, it did close with the bittersweet hope that discourse was possible and could be continued next year.

I thank you for your attention and commend you to this worthy work.

Systems-Centered Approaches

In this section a reader has an opportunity to get thoughtful, concise views of the interrelation of individual members and the social fabric of group systems. We chose these papers because we felt that each has a distinctive way of reflecting something of its writer's core assumptions about the nature of those relations.

Core assumptions in a theory of the group as a system include the assumption that a group's component elements influence one another, as well as the entire functioning group. Another core assumption is that a therapy group is a system of systems, with some suprasystems holding the group, as in agency practice, and subgroup constituents. These premises carry enormously wide implications and applications to social science theory as well as to therapy. No one is more a proponent of this distinctly social view and its distinctly personalist application to group therapy than Dr. Agazarian. Here she offers an excellent summary of her mature view of a group therapy that is not analytic/expressive but rather is directive.

Dr. Agazarian is not surpassed in having very thoughtfully created her comprehensive system of premises and practices in group treatment. Here some critical views of her SCT thinking, not often seen in publications, are offered. Dr. Aledort offers a theory of therapy that presents the therapist as a vigorous organizer of elements in a whole group. Dr. Aledort has clearly indicated his differences in approach with her work that he finds here, as he has in national conference workshops. Dr. Agazarian has said that hers is not an analytic group therapy; Dr. Aledort stresses the importance of including analytic ideas in doing the work. He puts work with transference relations at the center of analytic group work. A therapist, in his view, needs to be a vigorous organizer of all group elements. He puts transference relations with him at the center of group work.

In my critique, I call attention to the consideration that on the one hand Agazarian appeals to interpersonal influences in the work of subgroups, but on the other, she appeals to subjective experience at the expense of relations in the group and outside—she attends more to what is sometimes called a one-body psychology. I also call attention to the fact that the cultural-social-political world is an all-inclusive suprasystem; the depreciation of women in Freud's male-dominant world is an example of this suprasystem making a formative basis for his views, particularly his views of female sexuality.

Dr. Hopper describes the way that group analysis poses issues that personalities must come to grips with, such as important limitations and potentials for playing one's own part in contemporary culture. A person's subgroup identity in his/her group dynamics reflects the function therapy can have in her becoming a more mature citizen.

Dr. Skolnick's paper is probably one of the last of his written work to appear in print. His imagination ranges richly over references to topical issues as well as literary references. Here, in the service of therapeutic group events, he gives us a very stimulating glimpse into complex individual identity embedded in groups. In his view we are reminded how each individual needs to acquire the Lacanian symbolic register to be a social being.

Dr. Stiers offers us a dramatic analysis of what happens as a group becomes an increasingly adequate container of group feelings. He gives us a better way to understand the fate of groups dealing with explosive matters. His is a very simple and direct clinical demonstration that there are definable stages of group development. He gives us a better way to understand the fate of groups dealing with explosive matters: A group's capacity to contain explosive material is learned; it is not conferred by the therapist and is certainly not something that individual members bring already formed within them.

Stiers's paper gives specificity to the general idea that a therapy group develops by stages toward greater cohesion and therefore staying and holding power. Stiers also documents what I believe is the growth of conscious and unconscious love among members, which tempers reactions with empathy and stimulates members' acceptance of each other. Considerateness also grows, which makes members' comments to one another more acceptable.

For other recent readings in systems theory and object relations, a reader might see the following:

Kibel, H. D. (2005). The evolution of the Group-as-a-Whole and Object Relations theory: From projection to introjection. *Group, 29*, 139–161.

Kernberg, O. E. (2003). Sanctioned social violence: A psychoanalytic view, Part I. *International Journal of Psychoanalysis, 84*, 683–698.

Kernberg, O. E. (2003). Sanctioned social violence: A psychoanalytic view, Part II. *International Journal of Psychoanalysis, 84*, 953–968.

Reading these papers, I became increasingly aware that *group* development is a multisubjective situation that comes into being as a conjoint product and promise of therapy, as well as of reflectiveness and considerateness that amounts to conscious and unconscious love. Ogden describes an "analytic third subject" that grows and grows between the analytic pair, that exercises a background influence over the depth and extensiveness of their communication—a connection of *tested trust* that grows. So too we can imagine that a group creates a background multisubjective fourth subject that exists in members' shared mutual understandings and that exists nowhere else for those members or in any other group. This unique being-together is product and promise of the particular ways that these members have learned to interact. It exists inside other institutions, including perhaps the agency or practice wherein the group functions and, ultimately, in the institution of psychotherapy that our culture has evolved.

Sy Rubenfeld

Introduction to a Theory of Living Human Systems and Systems-Centered Practice

YVONNE M. AGAZARIAN

Introduction

The purpose of developing new concepts—new ways of thinking and seeing—is so that we can do things that we couldn't do in the world before we saw it through new eyes. Thinking "systems-centered" instead of "patient-centered" is an example of this.

In our role of therapists doing therapy systems-centered thinking "should" help us understand the world of psychology differently so that we can do things therapeutically that we couldn't do before—in individual therapy, or group therapy, or family therapy, or any one of the many specialized therapies.

Certainly applying systems-centered thinking to group therapy *did* help me see and do things differently as a group therapist. I came to see subgroups rather than individuals as the basic unit of the group-as-a-whole, and to focus on "system roles" rather than group member-roles as the most powerful and economical way to therapeutic changes for both the individual and the group.

Systems-centered thinking orients our understanding to the dynamics of systems so that we do not require of ourselves and of others changes that the state of the system makes it impossible to achieve. Sometimes we must change the larger system first before we can change others—or ourselves.

This paper introduces systems-centered thinking and its systems-centered practice.

The Nuts and Bolts of Systems-Centered Theory

I.   A system exists in an environment. The system of group, for example, exists in the group room!

II.   A system has boundaries. The system of group exists inside the boundaries of space and time. *Space boundaries* mark the threshold between the system inside and outside of the system: for example, group members come "in" to the circle to establish the group. *Time boundaries* differentiate between the past, present, and future of a system, both in real clock time and in psychological time. This is true, of course, whether the system under scrutiny is the system of a group, an individual, or the organization to which both belong.

III.   System boundaries are potentially permeable. Information can be transferred and sent across the system boundaries of the group, its members, and its subgroups.

IV.   System energy is contained within the boundaries of the system. How permeable the boundaries are, and what they are permeable to, determines how much energy is available for system maintenance and how much energy is available for work.*

V.   Systems have goals. The internal goal of every system is to survive and develop. The external goal of the system is the target of its work. Goals that are made explicit to the system are more likely to be reached.

Dealing With Difference

Systems survive, develop, and transform by integrating energy in the form of information—thus the systems-centered assumption that this is both the necessary and sufficient condition for therapeutic change. The assumption states that all living human systems survive, develop, and transform from simpler to more complex as a function of the discrimination and integration of differences—both the discrimination of differences in the apparently similar and the similarities in the apparently different.

Universally, difference is a maturing experience in that it requires taking apart the existing organization of information sufficiently to "take in" the difference and integrate it into a new organization that contains both the "old" and the "new" in a different form.

But difference is also dissonant and disorganizing. Introducing difference disequilibrates the system. When the system is in equilibrium, system energy is organized in the service of system goals. When difference results in dissonance within the system, the system energy is disorganized—and disorganized energy

---

* Information is equated with energy (Miller, 1978).

is disequilibrating and uncomfortable. Attending to the discomfort generated by differences can become more important than the group goals.

One way to reduce dissonance in the system is to create a subsystem (a system within a system) to contain the difference and wall it off behind an impermeable boundary that makes sure that the "difference" stays inside. This can be a permanent or a temporary solution: permanent results in fixation in the process of maturation and the loss of potential resources, temporary is the solution that a system employs until it has matured sufficiently to be able to take in and integrate the difference with less dissonance.

Another way to reduce dissonance in the system is to discharge it into the environment. Action crosses the boundary of the system influences the system's relationship with its environment. For example, the group can blame something in the environment, like the boss or the organization or the rules, rather than address the frustration that their leader has not solved their problems for them.

Another popular way of avoiding the task of integrating difference is to form stereotype subgroups by implicitly grouping members around gender, race, religion, status, etc., and maintaining the differences by developing one kind of communication pattern within the different groups, and another kind of communication pattern between the groups. These stereotype subgroups can be either a temporary or permanent solution. Another solution to maintaining the status quo is to create stereotype roles like scapegoat or identified patient, into which the unacceptable differences are projected and institutionalized.

Functional Subgrouping

SCT leaders deliberately discourage stereotype subgrouping: in which members join around the comfortably similar and differences are typically institutionalized or scapegoated. Instead, SCT leaders promote functional subgrouping, which requires members to subgroup around similarities before differences are addressed. Functional subgrouping also promotes building on common experience rather than using the defensive "yes, but" kinds of communication in which members appear to be building on what the last member said but are actually preempting the conversation. In an SCT group, when members introduce explicit differences, the therapist intervenes and says something like, "That is an important difference. Could you hold on to that, and not forget it, and bring it in later after we have finished exploring the issue that we are talking about now?"

All subgroups spontaneously come together around similarities and separate around differences. The work of the systems-centered therapist is to transform stereotype subgroups into functional subgroups so that the process of discrimination and integration that leads to the development and transformation of the system can occur. This requires maintaining the permeability potential of the system boundaries. It is characteristic of systems that they open boundaries to information and close their boundaries to noise. One form of noise we have already discussed: when differences are too different to be integrated.

Another form of noise is the ambiguities, redundancies, and contradictions in the communication that make it difficult for clear information to get across. The systems-centered therapist reduces this form of noise whenever possible. For example, when communication becomes redundant, the "content too similar," then the therapist points out overlooked differences. When the group becomes too contentious or too contradictory, then the therapist points out overlooked similarities.*

The Work of the Systems-Centered Therapist

All of the above issues are the material for systems-centered interventions. Generally, behaviors that serve as driving forces in a group are those behaviors that are conflict free, and generally behaviors that serve as restraining forces are conflicted behaviors, or manifestations of conflict. It is up to the systems-centered therapist to recognize the difference, and to encourage the group members to experience the differences for themselves.

The easiest way to reduce resistance to the driving forces that move toward the goal is to weaken the restraining forces. In systems-centered theory, defenses and symptoms are interpreted as restraining forces. Thus somatic symptoms, character defenses, tactical defenses, and the cognitive and physiological responses to anxiety are all understood as barriers in the journey toward the goal.

Defensive restraining forces are weakened in a prescribed order. Readiness is established by targeting the specific defenses that are generic to the phase of development that the group is in. Thus by weakening the anxieties that are generated by anxiety provoking thoughts in the flight phase, members regain their ability to use their minds to test reality. By discriminating between tension and frustration in the transition phase between flight and fight, members discover the energy in frustration, separate from the constriction of tension, and begin the work of regaining their physical and emotional relationship to their body. This in turn prepares the members to recognize depression as the retaliatory impulse turned back upon them, and to discriminate between containing the impulse and acting it out.

Defenses themselves develop from simpler to more complex. Thus, when each defense is weakened in the appropriate context, the very work of weakening the simpler defense lays the groundwork for weakening the more complex defense that follows. In the systems-centered approach this is called the hierarchy of defense modification. One of the goals of the systems-centered leader is to "train" the group to recognize and monitor its own restraining forces in each phase of group development and to make the discrimination between the

---

* Shannon & Weaver (1964) hypothesized an inverse relationship between noise (ambiguities, contradictions, and redundancies) in the communication channel and the probability that the information it contains will be received.

defense and what is being defended against discrimination fundamental to systems-centered practice.

Another difference in the systems-centered orientation is the avoidance of interpreting "why." The systems-centered therapist deals with "how" communication occurs, NOT "what" is implicated by the content of the communication. The underlying assumption is that as members reduce the noise in their own communications and can express and hear themselves more clearly, they themselves come to an understanding of their own dynamics without interpretations from the therapist. When this occurs, insight is experiential rather than cognitive.

It is certainly helpful to listen to the content of the communication as a diagnostic implicit in group goals and subgroup voices, but the work of the systems-centered therapist is not to address the group content but to influence the process of how the content is communicated. A focus on process deemphasizes making clinical interpretations about what is being communicated or about the person communicating. It is the nature of communication that transactions across boundaries are the intervening variable that the systems-centered therapist influences. And there are some systems-centered guidelines for doing this.*

Subgrouping and the Dynamics of Splitting, Containment and Projective Identification

Certain dynamic constructs such as "splitting," "containment," and "projective identification" are dynamically equivalent to both systems-centered and object relations theory. From a systems perspective, these constructs are applied, not only to the individual, as they are in object relations theory, but also specifically to the subgroups of the group-as-a-whole. Subgroups are the subsystems that contain the splits that occur naturally around differences from the similarities. "Splitting" is the both the basic stabilizing mechanism by which differences are "contained" in the system and also the dynamic that permits the work of integration is done.†

---

* Some of the techniques of systems-centered practice are: The hierarchy of Defense Modification; The fork-in-the-road between the defense and what is being defended against; The Force Field of driving and restraining forces; Developing the member, subgroup, and group-as-a-whole system perspectives as an alternative to "taking things just personally"; and functional subgroup.

† The system's subgroups then interact with boundaries that are relatively closed to communication transactions that carry projected information until the general system has matured sufficiently to reintegrate it. This is seen in the group in a scapegoating communication pattern when the boundaries to the information are being maintained as closed, and in the form of a communication pattern to deviant when the boundaries are permeable.

Splitting in this sense is in the service of the maturation process of the system, which is to remain in a viable equilibrium while it interacts with its environment and develops secondary goals. The functions of splitting, projection, and denial are seen as potentially maturational functional in that they are mechanisms by which differences are isolated and contained in a subsystem within the system until, through further maturation, they can be integrated.

The process of functional subgrouping is central to the systems-centered method and capitalizes on the natural tendency of systems to split two sides of a conflict. In a systems-centered group, splitting conflicts and containing them at the group-as-a-whole level in functional subgroups is the deliberate technique for managing the developmental discriminations and integrations.

Subgrouping requires the group members to make the splits conscious, to bypass ambivalence, and to work on one side or another of the conflict. By containing and exploring both sides of the issue, the system does not have to bind its energy defensively or discharge it into the environment but can contain it in functional subgroups while the work of crossing the boundary between fantasy, wishes, fears, and actuality is done.

The purpose of systems-centered therapy is to increase the ability to keep frustration generating conflict contained within the system-as-a-whole or a subsystem structure, rather than acted out in repetitive, defensive, or stereotypical ways. Members in systems-centered groups are encouraged to understand how the defenses relate to the management of frustration, with the goal of tolerating frustration as a natural process for which neither the self, the situation, nor another is to blame.

Although splitting and projective identification are typically labeled pathological defenses, from the perspective of group-as-a-whole system theory, "splitting" and "containing" are deemed to serve as fundamental mechanisms in maturation. They are mechanisms that "store" information in a subsystem under specific vicissitudes of the normal maturation process. When information is too contradictory, ambiguous, or redundant for the system to integrate into its present organization, the system "splits off" that part of the information and projects it into a subgroup container.

A good example of the kind of work entailed in learning how to "contain" frustration occurred in a systems-centered training group. The group with great commitment was struggling to contain their frustration at how difficult group work is—a frustration that was increased by my asking the group to explore the experience of containing their frustration without finding an object to blame. They said, "I don't understand what you mean by 'contain the hatred without an object'" and "How can I be this angry without either hating you or this group or myself?" Just at that moment, the telephone, usually switched off during the group, rang. There was an instantaneous roar of laughter at just how intensely, and with what relief, everybody instantly hated the telephone. Almost immediately afterward came insight: "I need a home for my hatred." "Now I understand why I hate my mother / my parents / my boss / you!" "Now I understand what you mean when you say that if you don't 'contain' frustration, the hatred is fixating!"

Phases of Group Development

Systems are made, not born. In the systems-approach to the phases of development in group psychotherapy, the group is not left to develop naturally while the therapist "contains" the process and judiciously interprets it. Rather, the dynamic process forces are deliberately exploited, certain group behaviors are deliberately promoted, all dynamics, however primitive, are legitimized as primary experience requiring organization, and a problem-solving system is deliberately created so that the work of therapy is done by learning how to do the work of therapy that is appropriate to the developmental context.

From the perspective of object relations theory, which is essentially oriented toward individual dynamics, it is useful to know the phases of group-as-a-whole development and the systems-centered framework of functional subgrouping as the treatment context for the individual's characteristic relationship pattern.

It is important to discriminate between the power/control and intimacy phases of a developing group, if one is to help members to join a developing group "in phase." The loss of an apparently appropriate new member may well bewilder a therapist who does not "match" the member to the developing group phase. For example, insight for individual members into individual dependency and counterdependency; relationships to authority; and work with their underlying depressive dynamics occur most easily in the first phase of group development, and insight into individual issues of interpersonal closeness and distance; love addiction; loneliness; alienation; despair; and work with the underlying schizoid paranoid dynamics occur most easily in the second phase of group development. When individual work is "in phase," members in the group spontaneously access memories and feelings that serve as stimuli that are relevant to the general work and specific to their own. Thus, groups provide the context in which individual developmental issues are revisited. Group members mature as the group learns to work and to love and to play!

System development is isomorphic (mirroring in structure, function, and dynamics) at the level of the group, the subgroup, and the individual member—and the resolution of the vicissitudes innate in each developmental phase of the group-as a whole potentiates the resolution of the developmental vicissitudes of the individual. Thus what was a past fixation or irresolution for the early phases of individual development is re-reworked in the present resolution of group development.

In systems-centered therapy, the therapist transfers his technical resources to the group as fast as the group is able to use them. Thus the first step in therapy requires the group to recognize its defenses, and make them ego alien to the group-as-a-whole, though supported, whenever necessary, in a balancing subgroup.

In making the transition between developing theory and putting it into practice, I found that I was changing, not only my approach, but also the way I used language in the group. I found myself dropping certain words out of my therapeutic vocabulary and substituting the words that reflected some of the basic changes that systems-centered work required. As systems-centered therapists, we are no longer problem oriented. We find ourselves depathologizing, humanizing, and legitimizing universal dynamics. We find ourselves observing and communicating an understanding of group members' difficulties as inherent to the human condition rather than personal.

It became increasingly clear that in the early phases of group development almost all leader communications, however descriptive, are experienced as superego injunctions, and interpretations of unconscious motive vastly increase group anxiety, defensiveness and dependency. That when the members imitate the intervention style of the leader (as all members do before they gain autonomy in the group) their interpretative style is not only an identification with the aggressor but also an effective method of turning communication into ammunition in the power, control, and status fights of the first phase.

It also became clear that for us as clinicians, the human tendency to discharge hostility in punitive language finds an easy expression by pathologizing normal group system dynamics—for example, the tendency to question the unconscious motives underlying behavior rather than to observe the function of the behavior in terms of system development. Or, for another example, dealing with the "identified patient" and the "scapegoat" in terms of unconscious motivation of the individual, or as an interpersonal repetition compulsion for the pair. This will of course have a very different outcome from understanding that these are roles created by the group to split off and contain, through projective identification, difference that the group is not yet ready to integrate. There is danger of developmental fixation if creating subgroup roles for deviants becomes the solution to differences in the group; or worse, for the therapist. True enough that for the individual system the role is a function of a repetition compulsion. True enough these roles are a function of interpersonal role suction. However, insight into individual or interpersonal dynamics may be beneficial to the individual systems but will not help the group-as-a-whole or its subgroups to identify what aspect of developmental dynamics is being denied, repressed, and projected.

It seems to me that in the clinical field we are increasingly paying attention to how we tell the difference, in our work in therapy, between when we address issues that are generic to treating human ills, and when what we address are iatrogenic, regressive, or defensive constellations elicited by our treatment context and methods. In other words, when is our practice a function of our own rationalized projective identifications that require human containers for the differences that we and our society cannot bear, and when is it a function of enabling us to cross the boundaries between our different human systems so that we can work together toward our group goals? I am suggesting that looking at our work through systems eyes, and understanding the immutable influence of phases in the development of human group systems, may be a step toward this important discrimination.

References

Miller, J. (1978). *Living Systems.* New York: McGraw-Hill.
Shannon, C. E., & Weaver, W. (1964). *The Mathematical Theory of Communication.* Urbana, IL: University of Illinois Press.

Some Comments on the Similarities and Contrasts Between Dr. Agazarian's Systems-Centered Therapy and Dr. Aledort's Therapist-Centered Group Psychoanalysis

Stewart L. Aledort

These comments reflect the observations of an active observer during the first phase of the "educational process" in SCT, lead by Dr. Agazarian, at a 4-day conference at the National Group Psychotherapy Institute in June 1995. In our work Dr. Agazarian and I are powerful leaders who demand the group's constant gaze as a way to invoke powerful, early regressive transferences almost immediately. I assume that we both implicitly agree that, in the beginning, there is an enormous potential for the group to regress around a preoedipal mothering figure. I feel that both of us encourage this regression in a very similar fashion. Both of us demand eye contact and work with the bodily feelings. We both work individually with the patients while the others are either in subgroups waiting and pairing and gazing, or, in my case, are all looking at me work with one member as a subgroup of two. I encourage all the other members to look at us work. We are both searching for the good and bad fits between the patient and the therapist. Dr. Agazarian will keep working with one member until there is relief from strong somatic feelings, without explanation and mentation. I wonder if this is similar to Bion's admonition of the therapist's need to be without memory and desire. Dr. Agazarian clearly drives the regression to early symbiotic somatic experiences on a one-to-one basis, while the other members look and introject the symbiotic experience. I ask patients how they want me to fit with them so we can do the tough work ahead of us. I ask them to gaze at me and not at others for a long first phase, which can last up to 6 to 9 months.

The beginning group coalesces around the early symbiotic experiences that provoke excitement and other strong affects like hate and love. These intense feelings are called up in response to the power of the merger experience with its awesomeness, yearnings, delights, and terror. Dr. Agazarian doesn't want words and thoughts from her members, only feelings in the body, which drive the regression deeper into the sole confines of the body ego and its formless self.

In Dr. Agazarian's demonstration group, following this symbiotic merger, the participants shared fantasies of animals running wild, and they focused in fantasy on the animals' delicious bodies and their impulses. I think this reflected the excitement of the discovery of the body still within the confines of the preoedipal good-mother dyad. The body magnificent with its power, passion, and need to move and explore took to the fore. At this point the demonstration group had to end with the participants in various stages of euphoria and excitement. Many of the outside observers were filled with anger and envy at having to be alone with their own bodies, but along with the relief that they weren't in the demonstration group. The problem with these first-phase demonstration groups is that you don't see the middle phases and therefore have to fantasize the rest.

I've tried to describe the similarities in the beginning stages of our groups as charismatic leaders. Because of our crucial and central position within the group, Dr. Agazarian and I both work very hard to control the boundaries and any acting out within the group. We each assume responsibility for containing and metabolizing the powerful feelings of awe, excitement, power, idealization, hate, and love that are thrust into us. In addition, we have to pay special attention to how we may inoculate our groups.

Dr. Agazarian and I would both agree that the early phases of the group, which is shaped almost exclusively by the therapist's theories and actions, has an enormous impact on the rest of the group's history and its outcome. What do we each bring to the groups that can hinder or facilitate character growth and successful terminations? What do we each bring to our groups that will either allow new patients to fit in easily or with difficulty? The questions appear crucial for us to answer in due course.

Dr. Agazarian and I do part ways in our theories and in our understanding of fantasies, acting in the group, transference, and interpretation. I believe strongly that each patient must have room to exhibit and act in his own personal drama that he had come to get repaired either through the fantasy of making the drama more efficient or really changing the internal mechanisms of the dramas. Therefore, my patients will engage in all kinds of dramas such as scapegoating, isolating one member, power plays, sadistic and masochistic behavior, seductions of all kinds, and various forms of narcissistic manipulations. I feel this is essential to the work and exploration that lead to character change. Dr. Agazarian seems to believe that these actions and dramas are antithetical to character work. She seems to try her best to erase from the group genetic dramas and will actively stop patients who are trying to engage in it, rather than let it happen and deal with it. As a result of this control of what people can bring in, there feels to me to be a homogenizing effect at the beginning of the work. I can't comment on the later phases of her work, as I have not observed it. This effect is explained by Dr. Agazarian as the educative process and behavioral condition that she feels patients need in order to do the rest of the work, which is defense modification. I'm concerned that this educative process inhibits patients' capacity in later stages to explore, without limitations, the dramas of their personal lives both in and out of group. I suspect that the members of the group don't really notice what they may have given up to be in the symbiotic merger phase, with both Dr. Agazarian and the pairing subgroups.

Dr. Agazarian doesn't seem to believe in the value of interpretations, as she sees them as projections without facts behind them. Explanations of people's dramas and where they came from are crucial in my work and I believe can clearly serve as another adjunct to the containing functions of the analyst. Dr. Agazarian and I disagree strongly about this. I think interpretations that work have to first derive from metabolized and digested projections, genetic and somatic facts, and exploration of the early, highly-cathected organizing fantasies of the patient's relationship to group members and the leader. The analyst must then time the interpretation to arouse a good fit in the ongoing developmental phase, which is being addressed in the analytic work. This timing hopefully will shift a bad fit to a good fit and begin to neutralize the aggression and eroticism that have been part of the bad passionately held narcissistic fit.

For example, a new patient in my three-times-a-week group was continually mesmerizing and seducing the group with his soft, pied piper voice. The group consistently got aroused and terrified about this invitation to merge through his voice with him. After many experiences of this kind an interpretation was made that clarified for the patient and group the problem they were having with each other. I explained that because of the patient's history of being terrified to merge with his psychotic and sadistic mother he still needed to experience a sense of merger that he could control. His invitation, however, was filled with his mother's aggression and sadism and the group was reenacting for him his intense fear of being vacuumed up into his mother's frightening insides. He was trying unsuccessfully to smooth out the aggression by being so soft and seductive, yet he still couldn't neutralize the aggression. An important good fit occurred for him and the group and the movement forward for the patient has been remarkable in terms of his recollection of lost memories and affect and his increasing attempts to put into words, instead of action, his need to be close and be attached. The group can now safely look at their own needs to merge and how they try to neutralize their own internalized aggression.

When an interpretation is made and then leads to movement to a new level of psychic development, I assume that the interpretation acted like a good-enough mother in that it neutralized the irritability and aggression that coincided with a bad fit that the patient was reenacting and reliving. I think this good fit of the interpretation at the right developmental level and phase explains the power of the interpretation. A good interpretation acts like a healthy rapprochement experience.

I think the facts of a patient's genetic history as well as his own experience with the group are not just quantifiable bits of data but can also represent a peek into organizing fantasies that he has used all his life or at times in his life. It can represent induced affective experiences through transference experiences as well as projective identification experiences. So I think we need a broader definition of the facts than Dr. Agazarian currently uses.

I don't believe that the patient always knows what is best for him, especially around when to terminate the treatment. Dr. Agazarian seems to have said that the patient can unilaterally determine the termination of the treatment. Many patients terminate treatment when they are feeling better but also when they do not want to take the next step, especially in the further exploration of the narcissistic underpinnings of character formation (the Omnipotent Child). I ask the patient to keep working further when I suspect, from the data collected so far, that there are many narcissistic entitlements that are lying hidden that need to be analyzed to ensure further character change.

I have expressed many differences and similarities and still have many questions for Dr. Agazarian and her work to answer. I would like to know what she does with the analysis of the fantasies generated through the subgrouping. This seems to me fertile ground for enormous work. I would like to know what she does with the entitlements that narcissistic disorders promote. I put enormous energy into analyzing and working through the narcissistic issues at each developmental phase and have trouble with Dr. Agazarian's avoiding the term completely and reducing all narcissistic issues to the patient just "taking things personally." Many narcissistic defenses and entitlements act as stabilizers of the "self." I would like to know what Dr. Agazarian does with organized fantasies, with the organized "omnipotent child" states, and with the anxiety of excitement. Further, I am interested in understanding Dr. Agazarian's parameters for character change in therapy groups, and her thoughts about the impact of the preverbal push to be verbal on the genesis of the repetition compulsion. Lastly, I would like to know the cost to Dr. Agazarian and her group when she transitions from being the central character in the drama to the more peripheral one. My recent experience with Dr. Agazarian intellectually excited me and inspired me to write, and for this I thank her and look forward to our working together in San Francisco in February 1996.

Panel Discussion of Dr. Agazarian's Presentation of Systems-Centered Group Therapy

SY RUBENFELD

Hannah Decker (1991), a historian, provides a remarkable account of the Viennese world of Freud and of Dora, Freud's patient in his time-honored "Fragment of a Psychoanalysis." Decker begins a chapter with this: "Dora's psychopathology was constructed on a foundation laid by a willful father and an angry mother and buttressed by a patriarchal society and an anti-semitic world."

Here we have a statement of a systems hierarchy: intrapsychic subsystems, the oedipal multisubjective, and the suprasystems of the time. It seems a fitting preface to the world of ideas, creatively used and anchored by Dr. Agazarian in her systems theory, generated since the case that Freud labeled "merely a case of petite hysteria"—a label that the cultural suprasystem of his time and place had for the psychic effects on women of its blind disempowerment and devaluation of them.

Dr. Agazarian has developed one the most articulated theories of group process and therapy, and gifts us with stunning insights as she goes along, such as "The tragedy of stubbornness is that it saves inner life and on the other hand makes that inner life impossible to live." Her translation into activist use of symbolic objects common to psychodynamic theory, with splitting as an example par excellence, is remarkable in its crafted originality.

The very detail of her project—the compendium of strategy and tactics she employs in her modeling and demonstration, the density of her abstract theorizing pages in her paper in *Ring of Fire* (1994)—fairly invites critical challenge here [in the Institute conference], to which she must construct replies, to which some including myself find that she has too many answers. This is more stressful than ironic-funny: the contained containing the contending container. Indeed Bion's (1970) ideas of the uneasy relations between a container and the originality of its contained may be the best way we have for understanding the state of inspiration and opposition that systems-centered theory and therapy (hereafter referred to as SCT) incites (excites?) in its milieu of psychodynamic group therapy.

My observations/discriminations/reservations follow.

1.

Macario Giraldo of our faculty has made the observation here that SCT is premised on psychoanalytic ego psychology and classical drive/structure theory as distinct from Fairbairnian, object-seeking theory. I found this an enormously useful discrimination. It put into perspective, for instance, Marvin Skolnick making the distinction, in his [Institute conference] colloquy with Dr Agazarian, "I find it better to connect with the other and then understand" in contrast to her "I find it better to connect with self and then go out."

Ogden says, "Each person is destined to remain outside of himself (alienated from self) insofar as the other has not given him back to himself by recognizing him." I believe that SCT might say that each person gives herself back to herself by recognizing herself in the other—that is, in the same or another functional subgroup. Personal observation and introspection would support this. SCT appears however to try to bypass or finesse 50 years of relational theory and therapy grounded in it. We have what appears to be a contradiction or a notable paradox, in SCT: a highly sophisticated group therapy which, considered apart from its social systems theory, relies primarily on a one-body psychology.

2.

That this is a problem becomes clear in considering SCT in relation to self psychology. Self psychology in essence is a view of what happens in one person in the presence or absence of empathic attentions and actions by another or others. It is fundamentally a relational, transactional theory and treatment approach. Agazarian states, from the standpoint that defenses are part of the ego apparatus, "Either respect the defenses or respect the person." I believe a self-psychologically oriented group therapist might reply that confronting a person in a way that might seem dismissive toward his defenses runs a great risk of being experienced as disrespect of him as a person.

The problems of self defect—that is, the vulnerability of self to disorganization through lack of internalized selfobject function—cannot be experienced by the therapist and group members except in interaction. In self psychological theory, projective attributions to others are considered evidence that the self is not experiencing an empathic response and is experiencing fears of impending breakdown in self-functioning. These projections have to be dealt with in some way so as not to undermine development in beginning SCT, as in any beginning of a therapy group. In SCT, however, they are managed out of the way, rather than worked with as signs of a self losing function in its awe before a new group. This kind of intervention runs the risk of a person feeling disrespect and then avoiding a further sense of injury through compliance.

SCT's teaching and then management of functional subgrouping promises powerful empathic experience and support. Members of the same subgroup, in offering their elaborations on kindred self experiences, should alleviate suffering alone, and often seem to. This behaviorally managed exchange of similar self states may be sufficient; only therapist use and evaluation in practice of the model can answer the question.

3.

The use of the phrase "behaviorally managed" above was deliberated because it is a loaded term. Many psychodynamic therapists feel besieged by managed behavioral therapies, not only because of threats to livelihood in the current environment but also because of the threat to a treatment outlook that receives, encourages, and responds to what is spontaneously expressed—as old an idea as free association. The very systematization that looks toward more efficient thera-peutic management, the explicit and superior demonstration by Dr. Agazarian of SCT, has invited reservations [expressed in the conference] that the unconscious cannot be controlled and that training and management of group members is not psychoanalytically oriented therapy. (Agazarian informally communicated that she does not consider SCT an analytic group therapy.)

One reply, it seems clear, could be that SCT prepares members more effi-ciently to be self-exploring and authentically expressive in later stages of develop-ment. Indeed that seems to be the whole point of the project; Agazarian reports this regarding an advanced SCT group. But can such means, instructing members as to what to do and not do, bring about ends of individuation and personal free-dom that are held forth for therapies that work from the first with what persons present in their own ways? I offer this question as one way to state the untrusting (not the welcoming and excited) side of the container's relation to the contained.

4.

A last reservation: As Agazarian has observed, system is a construct and is not there unless you look for it. Its use in SCT is manifestly powerful, i.e., tying many diverse phenomena meaningfully together. The value of the abstraction should not mislead into the mistake that a person is a system; just as, when Agazarian speaks of vectoring one's energy it should be clear that this refers to directing one's intentions: Vector and psychological energy are both constructs. My con-cern here is about the covert appeal of SCT, outside its intrinsic value as explana-tion and treatment method, in a technology-driven culture. The obvious analogy is to Freud's machine model in the industrial era in which he made psychoanalytic metatheory (as in his concepts of libidinal energy and defense mechanism).

5.

None of the above is to gainsay my gratitude and judgment about Agazarian's contributions in SCT. Her theory and technique of subgrouping, ensuring that a person is not left alone in his suffering, is a significant creation, at once profoundly informed and compassionate. Her delineation of group development phases open up better managing of group process. Her challenges to intellectualizing, "mind reading" as a means to smuggle in projective conjecture about another, and other defenses are clear. Her advice to therapists is very thoughtful: Do not flee from compassion into harshness or from sadistic feeling acted out in helping and solving. Standing on her grounding in information theory, she values and fights for the information in feelings against a prevailing therapeutic culture that fairly worships and overvalues the benefit of their enactment. I have been enlightened in ways that I shall use and assimilate still further.

Summary

This discussion discriminates between relational theories in general and the ego psychology used in SCT. Implications of this difference may be seen in the requirements that self theory seems to put on therapist action and modeling for members. Tensions generated between SCT and prevailing therapeutic culture are viewed as between directive and more receptive therapist reactions to members. A caution is raised about concretizing SCT concepts, and about SCT's latent appeal, outside its inherent merits, to the current technologizing cultural climate. Strikingly original contributions and observations of Agazarian are noted.

References

Agazarian., Y. M. (1994). The phases of group development and the systems-centered group. In V. L. Schermer & M. Pines (Eds.), *Ring of fire*. London: Routledge.

Bion, W. R. (1970). Container and contained. In W. R. Bion (Ed.), *Attention and interpretation: A scientific approach to insight and interpretation in psychoanalysis and groups*. New York: Basic Books.

Decker, H. S. (1991). *Freud, Dora, and Vienna 1900*. New York: Free Press.

Kohut, H. (1984). *How does analysis cure?* Chicago: University of Chicago Press.

Ogden, T. H. (1994). *Subjects of analysis*. Northvale, NJ: Jason Aronson.

Group Analysis and the Study of Maturity

EARL HOPPER

The purpose of this article, which is based on parts of a series of lectures to students of group psychotherapy at the Washington School of Psychiatry, is twofold: to propose that the ability and willingness to take the role of "citizen" is a central element of maturation and maturity; and to illustrate this with examples from twice weekly heterogeneous groups of adults who meet for the purpose of psychotherapy. I have developed my argument in much greater length in *The Social Unconscious: Selected Papers* (Hopper, 2003a) and in *The Fourth Basic Assumption in the Unconscious Life of Groups and Group-Like Social Systems* (Hopper, 2003b), which contain detailed clinical material and extensive bibliography.

The classical Freudian model of psychosexual maturity emphasized the resolution of problems presented by biologically based stages of development. According to this model, the ability and willingness to love, have heterosexual intercourse, to have children, and to work productively and gainfully—and to have pleasure in doing so—are the main characteristics of a mature person: The sociopsychological properties of a person were regarded as "natural," rooted in the growth and development of the organism; and although social, cultural, and political factors might interfere with growth and development, they were not regarded as determinant. In addition to the fundamental shift of emphasis suggested by Fairbairnian, Kleinian, and Winnicottian notions concerning preoedipal development, equally important shifts were suggested by anthropologists such as Malinowski and Richards, social psychologists such as Maslow, and psychoanalysts such as G. Klein, Erikson, and Stack-Sullivan. Thus, biological determinism, on the one hand, and social and cultural determinism, on the other, were at the foundation of this neoclassical psychoanalytical model of personal development.

In contrast, for group analysts the sociality of human nature was axiomatic. They believed that psychic facts are preceded by both organic and social facts and that a "person" is a human agent who has both a body and a society. Therefore, it was essential to give more emphasis to the contributions of existentialism and the importance of political factors and political actions, that is, the ability and willingness to make choices and to exercise the transcendent imagination. In other words, the development and the maintenance of mature hope was essential to the clinical project.

Group analysis was developed by S. H. Foulkes and by his colleagues James Anthony, the late Jim Hume, Lionel Kreeger, the late Tom Main, Malcolm Pines, the late Robin Skynner, and Stuart Whiteley, and it continues to be developed by the second generation of group analysts: Harold Behr, Dennis Brown, Liesel Hearst, Meg Sharpe, the late Louis Zinkin, and myself, among others. The group analytical perspective originated during the 1930s in the work of Erich Fromm, Karen Homey, and other members of the sociocultural school of psychoanalysis in Germany and Austria and in the sociology of Norbert Elias and his colleagues in the early Frankfurt School of Sociology.

The importance of the existentialist/political perspective in group analysis can be traced to a little-known paper, first drafted in the 1930s, called "The Revolutionary Character" by Erich Fromm (1963). (Personally, I rather like the title, but I can see that some people might be bothered by the connotations of "revolution" and especially by the fact that the book in which it was later published was entitled *The Dogma of Christ.)* Fromm writes:

> "The Revolutionary Character" is someone who is identified with humanity, and therefore transcends the narrow limits of his own society and who is able therefore to criticize his or any other society. He is not caught in the parochial culture in which he happens to be born, which is nothing but an accident of time and geography. He is able to look at his environment with the open eyes of a man who is awake and who finds the criteria of judging the accidental and that which is not accidental according to the norms which are in and for the human race. (1963, p. 111)

By "revolutionary character," Fromm really means "the mature person" rather than a character type. He is suggesting a stage of development in which a person can be sufficiently detached to be able to take his social circumstances as problematic but sufficiently involved to be able to identify with them and to be affected by them and, in turn, to be willing to affect them. To reach a point whereby one can be compassionate, sympathetic, and empathetic, yet sufficiently detached to take a situation as problematic, is a great psychological achievement. An infant cannot do this. Human beings must *strive* to achieve this "balance," which indicates that a certain kind of maturity has been reached.

According to this perspective, that which is not "accidental" is that which is "rational," or at least which can be explained rationally, according to the laws of science, including the laws of social science. Thus, the mature person is one who is able to transcend the limits of his own particular background and, therefore, to reflect upon his circumstances, to take them as problematic, and to locate them within their historical and contemporary social context. Such a person is able and willing to think about his own psychic life and that of others, his own inter-personal community and that of others, and his own identity and that of others. Such a person will be aware of the relativity of social and personal ethics, even if ignorant of the technical language needed to discuss it, and will have considered the traditional free will/determinism problem, even if he has never learned that the idea that we must try not only to understand reality but also to change it was a Marxist, revolutionary idea.

The revolutionary character will be able and willing to take the risks involved in attempting to change the very social circumstances within which he has come to be able to think, to make judgments, to act, and to be creative. He will have developed the ability to withstand and even to make creative use of social resis-tance to "revolutionary" action. He will be confident that attacks on authority are not always an expression of unresolved oedipal struggles, just as attempts by those in authority to maintain the status quo are not always an expression of their sense of responsibility and probity.

"Maturity" includes the development of the willingness and ability to take the roles associated with the status of "citizen." Inevitably, this will also be a group phenomenon in that people cannot take such roles if they have not ensured that the status of a citizen is available, which is a political process. This point of view was influenced by the work of T. H. Marshall (1949/1963) who, in an attempt to develop the economist Alfred Marshall's discussion of inequality, argued that the institutionalization of the rights of citizenship offered a fundamental social unity that could ameliorate the effects of those inequalities that might have to be borne in any large, complex, modern society. The willingness and ability to take the roles of citizen and to ensure that such roles exist within a democratic society can be facilitated through what Foulkes (1964) termed "ego training in action." Certainly, the spirit of impersonal fellowship as a core element in *Koinonia* (de Mare, Piper, & Thompson, 1991) can be understood in these terms.

Group analysts would include this concept of the revolutionary character within the neoclassical model of "genital maturity," but for them the concept of a revolutionary character subsumes the concept of genital maturity. The therapeutic and analytical process should involve attempts to make the social unconscious conscious. Maturity requires the substitution of ego both for id and for society, culture, and political factors and forces, which is a process that should continue throughout life.

The clinical relevance of these ideas can be illustrated with description of aspects of the actions and feelings "achieved" by three members of my twice-weekly groups:

> **1.** A Black male nurse who had immigrated to London from the Carib-bean experienced great frustration and humiliation in connection with his work with colleagues who were members of the medical profession, especially those who were older, White, and English. However, slowly he

became more active in the politics of his profession and in his hospital. He initiated a new committee consisting of both medical and nonmedical personnel, and it seemed that this committee would do some good work in alleviating the anxious concerns that were interfering with the clinical work in his department. As he became more proficient in understanding other subcultures as well as his own, he recognized that his own worldview was problematic—that is, although it was valid, it was based on a number of dimensions of his life experience that were not shared by others. Eventually, he was able to adopt the folkways and styles of his colleagues, not in a conformist and compliant way, but in a realistic adaptation to his new circumstances. In his political activities within his hospital he conducted himself with determination and resolve but also with dignity and self-control, despite the usual pressures put upon him by his opponents, especially those in authority.

2. A middle-class Jewish woman, 32 years of age, was unable and/or unwilling to make relationships with men, although she longed to be in love, marry, and have children. She had a history of failed relationships—that is, although they started well, she always found fault with her partners and ended what had seemed to be very appropriate and satisfying relationships. Eventually, she acknowledged that when she thought about her vulnerable father, she thought about him as her "Jewish father" and connected this image with her inability to make relationships with Jewish men, whom she felt were "weak" and "feminine." This caused her some sense of confusion because she wanted to please herself as well as her parents, who wanted her to marry a Jew. She also acknowledged that she thought of herself as a Jewish boy or specifically as a Jewish son who felt herself to be a woman only in relationship to Christian men. Eventually she may recognize her desire to be mothered by the women whom she perceives to be behind the men in her life, but in the meantime she is in the process of discovering that it is possible to negotiate her own gender identity, although, for reasons of both biology and of sociology, not entirely as she pleases. She has begun to understand how her gender, class, and religious identities are completely intertwined and has maintained a relationship with a non-Jewish man who she feels to be a "motherly man." This relationship has lasted for 2 years. She is now 4 months pregnant.

3. A homosexual psychiatrist from the Continent wished to become a group analyst. He became convinced that homosexuality was a counterindication for acceptance for training by the Institute despite evidence to the contrary. Rather than confront the relevant committees and their perceived policies, he renounced his aspirations. He was unable to make use of the views offered by the other members of the group and myself that not only was he frightened to be judged and assessed by authorities whom he respected, but he was also terrified to learn more about how he used his homosexuality to defend against psychotic anxieties and to express his sadomasochistic desires. Following a prolonged period of hatred of another male candidate, he left the group at short notice. I was unable to communicate to him in a meaningful way that he was repeating his hatred of his "chosen" little brother, and his conviction that I preferred his brother to him, as would the Institute. I regard this as an example of a therapeutic "failure"—mine, ours, and his.

Implied in this perspective and in these illustrations of it, is a way of thinking about participation in groups of all sizes. For example, a group analyst would argue that a mature work group is based on the development and maintenance of the ability and willingness of the participants in the group to function as citizens of it and to guarantee one another's rights to do so. In contrast, Turquet (1975), from a group-relations perspective associated with the work of Dion and his colleagues at the Tavistock Clinic, argued that in large groups individuals are likely to experience a regression to the status of a "singleton" or of an "isolate" and then, if all goes well, progress to the status of a "membership individual" and eventually to that of an "individual member," and, hence, the development and maintenance of a work group is based on the emergence of "individual members." However, the concept of "individual member" is subsumed by the concept of "citizen," which is far more comprehensive and dynamic in its implications.

Another implication of the group analytical perspective is that the maintenance of an easy balance between involvement and detachment is essential to the therapeutic and analytical attitude, both in dyadic and in group work of all kinds. This balance is also important in the conduct of sociological research and organizational consultation, especially when based on participant observation (Elias, 1956). In fact, all patients should have a long-term experience of participation in small and large groups. Not only might they learn more about the social psychology of groups and group-like social systems, but they would also have an opportunity to resolve some of the specific anxieties associated with becoming a citizen. This is obviously important for students of group analysis, but it is also important, and perhaps especially important, for sociologists, on the one hand, and psychoanalysts, on the other. However, this requires that our Institutes form and maintain a policy to this effect and have the will to realize it, which is itself a product of a political process.

References

de Mare, P., Piper, R., & Thompson, S. (1991). *Koinonia*. London: Karnac Books.

Elias, N. (1956). Problems of involvement and detachment. *British Journal of Sociology,* 7, 226–252.

Foulkes, S. H. (1964). *Therapeutic group analysis*. London: Allen and Unwin.

Fromm, E. (1963). The revolutionary character. In *The dogma of Christ*. New York: Holt, Rinehart and Winston.

Hopper, E. (2003a). *The social unconscious: Selected papers.* London: Jessica Kingsley Publishers.

Hopper, E. (2003b). *The fourth basic assumption in the unconscious life of groups and group-like social systems.* London: Jessica Kingsley Publishers.

Marshall, T. H. (1963). Citizenship and social class. In *Sociology at the crossroads.* London: Heinemann. (Original work published 1949)

Turquet, P. (1975). Threats to identity in the large group. In L. Kreeger (Ed.), *The large group: Dynamics and therapy.* London: Constable.

On Identity as Multiple and Basic Assumption

Marvin Skolnick

> The mistaken and unhappy notion that a man is an enduring unity is known to you. It is also know to you that man consists of a multitude of souls of numerous selves.
>
> **—Herman Hesse**

> I look for the group I find myself—I look for myself and I find a group.
>
> **—Margaret Rioch**

It is unclear how many of us agree with these assertions. The phenomenon of multiple selves is usually regarded as pathological and delusional, warranting a psychiatric diagnosis. For most of us in a quiet moment of reflection, a dip into a stream of consciousness often produces an image of a stable unitary self. However, at a moment of conflict with others, a dip into the stream may well reveal a turbulence that muddies the image of a unitary stable identity. If one begins to trace one's sense of self from one social context to another, it may lose its sense of sameness and take on a protean quality that flows like Heraclitus's river. Reflecting on my own sense of identity, the first phrase that came to me was "I am who I am—to define me otherwise is to limit me." Embarrassed to notice a resemblance to pronouncements of the God of the Old Testament, I explored my identity, further reaching for self-definitions I thought more modest and sustainable.

Not to be identified as a member of a large group is to suffer the agony of disappearing, which is worse than being labeled in a limiting or insulting manner. I reluctantly settled on "old, White, middle-class Jewish American male psychiatrist." Then it occurred to me that even these straightforward definitions of identity are provisional and contingent on context. For example, in my consultations in a nursing home, I am middle-aged. In the synagogue, which I seldom visit, I am still a boy since I never was bar mitzvahed. At a Klan rally I am likely to be tagged as non-White. In a group in which status is afforded to victimhood, I might feel more connected to my Jewish roots and the Holocaust, while in a group in which status is afforded to knowledge, I might veer toward an identity more steeped in my CV and clinical professorship. I have seldom questioned my identity as a heterosexual, but to imagine myself in prison for a life term brings that aspect of identity into question. Even gender identity is somewhat provisional. In a group of male neighbors who eschew feelings and speak only about football, microbreweries, and fixing cars, I might feel out of place and push closer to my anima as a counterpoint to the prevailing animus of the group. Other dimensions of being less demographical, such as where I am on the smart-dumb, attractive-unattractive, and compassionate-cruel continuums, are even more contingent on the vagaries of the group process and context. Put in this way, identity can be thought of as a kaleidoscopic show between the ears rather than an entity. When what projects an individual's internal identity screen is compatible with the show on the screen of others, the group basic assumption is likely to be stable although it might support exploitation of subgroups. When what plays on identity screens is incongruent, a more unstable situation obtains in the group that could lead either to fragmentation or, through struggle, to a more differentiated level of development.

Despite the nature of identity as an unstable construct contingent on social interaction, the threat of loss of identity can stir the most intense passions and anxieties known to mankind. Kafka captures the precariousness of human identity in the "Metamorphosis." Without adequate recognition at work and at home of his human identity, the protagonist on awakening one morning discovers that he has transformed into a cockroach. In Milton's poem *Paradise Lost* we can identify with Satan, who would rather be his own man in hell than subservient in heaven. Many have been willing not only to kill but to die to preserve identity. To participate in a large group often evokes the intensely painful threat of loss of identity as though it is a possession like a wallet. The use of the pronoun "we" not infrequently provokes a recoiling by others and a chorus of "speak for yourself," while to be excluded from the "we" of the group can stir the deepest shame and anxiety. How can these paradoxes and apparent contradictions be understood? What bearing do they have on group relations work?

Homo Sapiens' Guilt

From an existential perspective the being of the human being is problematical. The very nature of consciousness of being situates us always on the brink of nonbeing. We are always in the process of becoming in which being and human identity must be constantly renewed in the face of the ever-present threat of nonbeing.

The tiger has a positive identity that unfolds without anxiety and labor, whereas the sapiens has to constantly struggle to create and sustain identity. The assumption that a good solid identity is achievable serves, like Bion's group basic assumptions, as a buffer against the unbearable anxieties inherent in our human condition as self-reflective, shame-filled, guilt-prone, and vulnerable mortal group animals. A human identity cannot be created or sustained in isolation. It is embedded in group process requiring both recognition and differentiation from others. Yet, to possess an identity is to feel that as a dancer one is separate from the dance. The illusion that one's identity is independent of group process must be built on deception. The tearing away from this illusion as with other basic assumptions can unleash violence and induce panic and disintegration anxiety, but sustaining it tenaciously can exact tremendous cost to truth, result in lost opportunities for development, and wreak destruction.

What factors influence a sense of identity? Generally human identity emerges out of an interaction with what Bolas has referred to as the personal idiom (spontaneous gestures arising out of genetic endowment of the individual), the mother, the family, the nexus of involvement with informal and formal groups, and the culture. As Turquet has emphasized, identity is dependent on the skin of the other. In other words, it is contingent on the presence of others experienced as "not me." From religious, national ethnic, class, gender, and age perspectives, each of us experiences "me" attributions and "not me" attributions. As part of our identifications with those with whom we feel joined, we project into a reservoir of mostly desirable or good qualities sustained by folklore, traditions, and mythography of past glories that we can call upon to introject, particularly during hard times, to bolster identity. In our collective identities we also share a receptacle in which we put bad, undesirable, or unintegrated qualities (projective identification into the "not me other"). In this receptacle also are memories of past traumas that fuel and justify our aggressive energies toward the denigrated or "bad" other.

Lichtenstein has suggested that aggression and the urge to dominate are more likely a function of the struggle to maintain identity than a basic instinct as Freud and Melanie Klein have maintained. Volkan, whose interests in these matters stem from his personal roots in the Turkish/Greek strife, has framed these issues in graphic and relatively jargon-free ways. He postulates "skins" or boundaries that are containers of our identity: one skin is the tight skin that fits snugly around the individual person, whereas another loose skin fits like a tent that contains those with whom we share our identity and keeps out those of whom are "not me" or "not us." The tight skin contains micro characteristics that differentiate us from our family members or close associates, and the loose-fitting "tent" skin contains more macro characteristics that differentiate us from people in other "tents." To further extend Volkan's metaphor, basic assumptions leaders can be thought of as poles that hold up the tent.

When either the tight skin or the loose skin is ruffled, the ongoing sense of identity is threatened with collapse. This threat to identity can occur on a personal level—narcissistic injury like the loss of a job or a loved one aging or participation in a group relations conference. It can occur on a macro level (e.g., the loss of territory, war, political or economic power). In Washington, D.C., for instance, the morning after a Redskin defeat a rise in irritability suggests significant second-skin damage. When what has been lost cannot be regained, a mourning process may ensue in which acceptance can lead to more mature integration at a less omnipotent depressive mode of being.

When traumas are not acknowledged by empathic others, when there is not a stable containing environment or access to justice, a successful mourning process is highly problematical. In fragmented or rigidly stratified societies or where cycles of destructive violence prevail, the mourning process is often aborted. This often leads to solidification in a paranoid schizoid organization in which defenses such as splitting, denial, and projective identification play a prominent role in the maintenance of good-enough identity. In the paranoid schizoid mode of experience, differences between self and other are accentuated. If the "other" begins to be experienced as too much like "me" through transactions across boundaries such as trade, negotiations, or participation in a group relation conference, then the dimensions of identity supported by paranoid schizoid mechanisms are put at risk; this may result in what seems on the surface to be a paradoxical recoiling and exacerbation of conflict when reconciliation and appreciation of shared interests seem imminent.

Lacan, a very creative and complex thinker, who like Bion had a tendency to disturb the universe, has made some very pertinent but unsettling contributions to the question of identity. From his perspective any solid, clear notion of individual identity is primarily falsity. In his view the first sense of identity arises out of mis-recognitions creating what he terms the domain of the imaginary. Lacan believed the image perceived by the young child in the literal mirror and the image of the self experienced in the gaze of the mother is confused with the actual self. In the case of the literal mirror this confusion is born out of the desire to be much more of an autonomous going concern than one actually is, and in the case of the image perceived in the mother's eyes it is the intoxicating desire to experience oneself as the desired embodiment of what the mother lacks. Thus the bedrock of identity, if one can call these illusions bedrock, come out of the desire to transcend vulnerability and dependence and the desire to be the object of the others desire. This inflation of identity creates an intense feeling, which Lacan terms *jouissance.* Capturing the deep paradoxes around the sense of identity, Lacan suggests that jouissance is both the joy in the gratification of being desired and the horror at disappearing as a self into the whirlpool of the other's desire. It is through the intrusion of a third party—the name of the father, or language—that the imaginary dyad is ruptured, thrusting the child into the prevailing culture as a group animal. It is the infiltration with language, which Lacan terms the "symbolic register," that humanizes and enables individuals to link with other individuals to form coherent mosaics like family and societal groups beyond the confines of the original dyad. Out of this process a sense of shared reality is constructed. Lacan differentiates between reality and the Real. Reality is the normative consensus symbolically coded in the language but is not what is Real, which is beyond the powers of human beings to comprehend or put into words. Words only point to the Real; they cannot capture it. Rather than biological instincts, Lacan asserts that it is the language that forms the core of the human psyche and structures the unconscious. It is the other dwelling within. From this perspective the so-called individual is not a cohesive whole but hopelessly divided between the culture dwelling within, a false identity born out of the imperative to conform to the desire of the significant others like mother, and a true self or subject that emerges only when an aliveness to desire arising from within moves the subject beyond the shelter of the imaginary and the socially constructed culture to the border of the Real. An important implication of this perspective is that different languages construct different realties and human beings who may process their experience differently at deep unconscious levels: When an individual speaks, who is speaking? How often do we hear ourselves or others mouthing religious doctrine, political ideologies, ethnic or nationalistic slogans, or TV commercials in what Lacan calls empty speech not connected to the center of the subject? To speak more fully as a subject entails falling into a gap where individual identity is experienced as problematical and an ongoing endless discourse with a deceptive other—an unconscious with it slipping and sliding signifies parapraxes.

Although this abbreviated summary of Lacan's thought is inadequate to convey his disorienting but rich contributions, I hope this effort will stimulate further interest in exploring how the Lacanian worldview might complement our complex Bionian perspective. For example, Bion's view that the group is experienced at the deepest level of the psyche as the mother suggests a possible intersection with Lacan's domain of the imaginary. The individual's propensity or valence to conform to the suction of the group basic assumption could be understood as at least partially driven by the desire to be desired by the mother group—that is, to provide at an unconscious level what the group needs to experience itself as complete. To apply Lacan's theory to group relations suggests that an ongoing exploratory discourse take into account the interplay of the domain of imaginary and the unconscious. Further, it would be necessary for the emergence of full speech within a group as an alternative to a group process that enthralls members and entraps them in a false mirror. Lacan puts a French twist on Margaret Rioch's question of whether she is herself or the group. Human relations and group relations do not confine themselves to the neat compartments of Euclidian geometry. Individual identity, group dynamics, and culture, like everything else that we can talk about, are social constructs that emerge out of intersubjective process that, like the Möbius strip, has no inside or outside. The dancer is inseparable from the dance.

Since Freud's original formulations, there have been sea changes in the dynamics of identity formation. Modern life, according to Lichtenstein, has made the illusion of a stable identity even more problematical. In this technologically shrunken, pluralistic world, instead of internalizing a homogenized, consensual, social, objectified reality through the parents and other significant agents of society, the individual today is confronted with a much more relativistic universe. There are now a multitude of ways to organize oneself, the other, and the world in terms of value, epistemologies determined more by one's momentary identification with an array of groups than anything approaching a stable consensus on what is social reality and what is legitimate authority. This relativism, ushered in by the what Nietzsche termed the "death of God," is highlighted by Liechtenstein's point that individual, ethnic, national, and religious identities have become increasingly unstable with the advent of scientific refutations of myths and folklore and increased permeability of boundaries between cultures. Science has also failed as a reliable compass to lead human beings to the Promised Land. Instead the 20th century, with its great scientific and technological achievements, has been the most destructive in human history. In this more complex world multiple realties are linked with multiple selves—each substantially different take on reality leads to a crystallization of a different self. In the increasingly intergroup nature of experience, the identities of individuals shift in accord with changing social context affecting both the distribution of wealth and power and the more unconscious interplay of projective and interprojective fields. Human relating and struggles around identity seem to become more baffling and contentious rather than less.

Sampson has introduced the notion of a neo-Marxist politics of identity and what he calls the absent standard. In his view, the ruling class or elite of a society impose their version of reality, morals, and values through a covert standard buried in the language that fortifies their identity, as privileged at the expense of others who are marginalized, intimidated, and silenced. From a Lacan Vertex, the symbolic register favors one subgroup over another. For example, the chain of signifier of *White* has positive connotations, whereas *Black* has negative connotations in the European and English languages. The culture and institutions of slavery and its offspring racism are obvious examples in which White identity subtly supported by the symbolic register is linked with purity and goodness while Black identity is linked with dark, sinister, and evil and thus denigrated, using interpretations of texts such as the Bible and science as authoritative support. The religious and literary canons are other subtle and sometimes not-so-subtle vehicles that institutionalize privilege and exploitation. For example, although Conrad in *Heart of Darkness* illuminated the abuses and exploitative practices of colonialists, Said points out in his book *Culture of Imperialism* that indigenous peoples were portrayed in Conrad's novels as primarily hapless victims without a culture of their own. Foucault has shown how what is accepted as truth in a society is intimately linked with the exercise of covert power in which those who don't conform are disciplined and punished.

When social process is dominated by paranoid schizoid mechanisms of projective and introjective identification, denial, and splitting, individuals and subgroups are more likely to be locked into dichotomized identities on the basis of trivial physical visible differences along the lines of superior-inferior, good-evil, competent-incompetent, master-slave, and sadist-masochist. To ensure a voice for everyone in the social discourse would seem like an obvious remedy toward creating a more just society. However, to bring about meaningful dialogue, according to Sampson, is much more difficult than it might appear. The right to speak is not enough. Loosening the canons to allow for consideration of multiple realties and perspectives is one rectifying path that the multicultural movement has stressed. Free speech must be joined to political power to have impact on institutions that support discrimination. Sampson stresses the importance of ferreting out the absent standard to make it available for deconstruction to level the playing field and make room for the standards of groups subject to discrimination such as women, homosexuals, and people of color. However, the assumption that there is identity within ethnic, racial, religious, or national groups and that they speak with one voice with one standard is false. Salman Rushdie is a dramatic example of the price an individual may have to pay who refuses to live within the constraints of an identity imposed from within his own religious and ethnic group. How to develop a discourse between people speaking presumably from different standards without deteriorating into a Tower of Babel is a challenge that Sampson does not address directly. A process is needed that imagines the possibility of a shared frame of reference out of which hate and fear can be transformed through discourse into broader and deeper understanding.

How do all these considerations about identity pertain to group relations and the exercise of authority? We frequently observe that who leads, who follows, and who dissents is determined as much by irrational unconscious process as by the dictates of the formal role of objective judgments about the quality of leadership. More consideration of the illusory nature of individual identity and its dynamics can enrich and complement our group basic assumption theory, which has little to say about the individual dimension of the dialectic between the group animal at war with his groupishness and the group. It is difficult to find spaces in our society to explore vital questions about how to maintain a good-enough identity as a human being without damming, marginalizing, or silencing others.

Keats speaks to the heart of such a process. He writes, "Do you not see how necessary a world of pains and troubles is to school intelligence and make it a soul? A place where the heart must suffer in a thousand diverse ways. This heart that suffers is the mind's Bible, it is the mind's experience, and it is the teat from which the mind or intelligence sucks its identity."

AK Rice Group Relations conferences should be ideal places to shed the armor of falsified identities to allow the heart to suffer on its way toward a more integrated sense of the relatedness of being. However, when as conference staff we clasp too tightly to our favorite identities as things in themselves rather than as evolving and devolving social constructs growing out of the group process, we join the resistance to the exploration of the process.

To design conferences with staff billed as all White, all Black, all Jewish, or all Christian, for example, in efforts to be creative or politically proactive, risks promoting repetitions of dichotomizing sadomasochistic relationships. Although some learning can occur from repetition and role reversals, the absence of a staff as an interpreting third makes fuller digestion of experience and movement from a paranoid schizoid organization less likely.

We are in a better state of mind to promote deeper exploration and learning from experience when we take up Bion's recommendation to enter the work without intention, memory, or desire. Bion was heavily influenced by Keats's belief that the poet, to be deeply receptive to himself, others, and the world around him, needed to develop a negative capability—"to be able to live in mystery and doubt without irritable reaching after fact or reason." Living in mystery about oneself is a crucial aspect of negative capability that allows for inscribing into the heart and the soul, the world, and others. Being an effective consultant in this regard is like being an effective post in that we allow the group to make of us what they will. By then, recovering from what Bion describes as the numbing reality of the group, we are able to contribute from our experience rather than prepackaged notion and serve as a model of learning from experience. If we define ourselves too strongly and defensively, this cannot happen readily or at all—and we become a model of important but less transforming identity politics.

In Whitman's "Song of Myself," he captures the negative capability of going to the depths of the ugliness and the goodness of the human soul on the way to affirming an identity not requiring a denigrated other: "Nor is it you alone who knows what it is to be evil I am he who know what it is to be evil I too knitted the old knot of contrariety blab'd, blushed, resented, lied, stole, grudg'd. Had guile, anger, lust, hot wishes I dared not speak was wayward, vain, greedy shallow, sly, cowardly, malignant the snake the hog not wanting in me the cheating look, the frivolous word the adulterous wish not wanting." Sampson speaks to a postmodern perspective that had its origin in the insights of Nietzsche, followed by Marx, Foucault, Derrida, and others, that knowledge and power are inextricably tied together in the most complex and seamless ways. I believe that this is true. At the bottom of the ugly and deceitful way we treat others and sometimes ourselves there is no simple solution that can bypass living in the labyrinths and the complexity. There is no quick and easy way to reverse injustice without inflicting more injustice.

As Lichtenstein asserts, we cannot sustain our identity as humans without constructing language, myths, traditions, and histories that are at least partially false or even delusional. However, particularly as group relations consultants, we must also be revolutionaries who are willing to keep one foot out of our provincial culture (tribe) into a more cosmopolitan (cosmos) space. In order to escape the dead end of fundamentalism, we need to not only stay open to the validity of the experience of others but also be ready to question the absoluteness of even our most cherished beliefs. Stephen, the protagonist of *A Portrait of the Artist as a Young Man*, was named after the Greek mythological builder of the labyrinth. He speaks in Joyce's coming-of-age novel to the challenge of the individual who in his fierce integrity finds himself alienated from every group—his family, his mother, the church, the English oppressors, and the fanatical Irish patriots; he realizes he must take a major part in creating his own identity if he is to retain his integrity but cannot do it in a vacuum. In his last entry before leaving home "to seek misfortune," he writes, "Welcome, O life! I go to encounter for the millionth time the reality of experience and to forge in the smithy of my soul the uncreated conscience of my race." If we are to enlarge the human trend to include everyone, there is much painful and frightening experience always ahead of us on the way to create a consciousness and a conscience that can celebrate different ways of being without denigrating the other.

Containment and the Threat of Catastrophic Change in Psychotherapy Groups

MICHAEL J. STIERS

Wilfred Bion's seminal work, *Experiences in Groups* (1961), is considered by many group therapists to be a classic study of group behavior (Eisold, 1985). Despite the influence of his early work on groups, practitioners frequently find his later writings (Bion, 1962, 1963, 1965, 1967, 1970, 1977) difficult to apply to group settings. Meltzer (1978) believes that this difficulty may be a result of the idiosyncratic features of Bion's writings and the high level of abstraction at which Bion writes. He feels that these characteristics of Bion's writing style make heavy demands on the reader trying to understand and follow Bion's line of thought. Yet, despite these obstacles, James (1981) believes that Bion's psychoanalytic writings are valuable, if not essential, to a fuller understanding of the phenomena we meet with in group psychotherapy. In recent years several authors (James, 1984; Grinberg, 1985; Resnik, 1985; Schermer, 1985) have begun to explore the linkage between Bion's psychoanalytic work and group psychotherapy.

The purpose of this paper is to discuss the relationships among four concepts: projective identification, container-contained, (Ps <—> D), and catastrophic change.

Projective Identification and Container-Contained

Melanie Klein (1946) defines projective identification "as splitting off parts of the self and projecting them into another person" (p. 108). She adds later that this results in a "feeling of identification with the other person because one has attributed qualities or attributes of one's own to them" (Klein, 1955, p. 58). Her use of the word "into" as opposed to "onto" is significant. Most defenses described in psychoanalysis are intrapsychic defenses—for example, repression, reaction formation, denial, and so forth. These defenses are what a person does to himself. A person using projective identification is not only attempting to rid his consciousness of unacceptable impulses but also attempts to induce experiences in another and simultaneously attempts to exert control over the other.

So we can say at this point that there are two functions of projective identification. The first function is to serve as a "defense" to rid the self of unwanted elements. The second function is as a "means of control" in relation to external objects.

Bion (1962), however, proposes a third function, which is as a form of communication. This notion is grounded in his concept of containment. Bion offers a model of container-contained (1945) as an extension of the concept of projective identification. The model is based on the notion of the mother as a container for the infant's projected feelings, needs, or unwanted parts. It indicates that the mother enters into an emotional relationship with her child through a particular state of mind called "reverie." In this state she can be open and ready to take in and reflect upon and modify what the baby projects into her. She then empathically conveys back to the infant the modified version of the projected feelings conveying a sense that these feelings are bearable and can have meaning. The modified forms of the originally threatening experience now can become a precursor to a thought that can be reflected upon and eventually integrated with other experiences. There can, however, also be a negative containment process, whereby the mother is not only unable to detoxify the infant's projected fears but adds her own primitive anxieties, returning the original projection as a bad object that can only lead to further attempts at evacuation by the infant.

Returning to the case of the good-enough mother-infant dyad, eventually the infant introjects a model of the thinking couple: an internal version of the container-contained relationship. The introjection of the container-contained relationship allows for a dialectic thinking process, which ultimately creates verbal symbols that serve as the containers in which experience (the contained) can be organized and reorganized symbolically.

Vicissitudes of Growth: Container-Contained and (Ps <—> D)

Bion (1977) states that in order to achieve psychological growth one must go through "stages of disorganization, pain, and frustration" because the process of learning inherently involves moments of internal disruption and moments of reintegration. He refers to these shifts in internal experience as the dynamic between paranoid-schizoid and depressive states of organization (Ps <—> D).

Bion describes the paranoid-schizoid level of internal organization (Ps) as an inner state of disorganization caused by a threat to the internal world coming either from external reality or the unconscious, with the resulting feelings of loss, anxious insecurity, persecution, and depression. This leads to use of the defensive mechanisms of splitting, dissociation, idealization, omnipotence, and projective identification.

The depressive level of organization (D), on the other hand, is a process of reintegration of the internal disorganization by the discovery of a selected fact, meaning an emotion or idea that gives coherence to what is dispersed and introduces order to what was disorder. However, this organization can only happen if the personality can contain the chaotic disruption of the paranoid-schizoid state enabling coherence to occur. Grinberg, Sor, and Tabak de Bianchedi (1977) therefore emphasize that in the formation and use of thoughts necessary for growth, both processes, container-contained and (Ps <—> D), operate together, and we cannot ascribe more importance to one than the other. Simply put, we are saying that the mind, as the container, needs to hold the new psychic data and its resulting turbulence (Ps) long enough to allow new patterns of thought and emotional coherence to develop.

If we state the above concepts differently, we can say that learning involves at least partial disintegration of what we know. This leaves us disorganized with the resulting feelings of loss, insecurity, persecution, and depression, because our container-contained is momentarily disturbed. That is, our symbolic representations or knowledge of the world cannot organize the new experience. We are forced to endure a state of confused "not knowing" waiting for a sense of cohesion to crystallize. This can be bearable if one has had a good enough history of object relations, where the mother engaged with the child in emotional encounters that provided container-contained experiences. Having had this, in most instances the individual can bear the impingement by unorganized sense and emotional stimuli without feeling unduly persecuted or depressed (Billow, 1986).

The Threat of Catastrophic Change

In line with what has been discussed so far, Bion (1967) suggests that some aspect of the personality is stable and constant (the container) and this part of the personality is the mechanism likely to contain emergent ideas that express new awareness of the reality of the self and the world. If this continuous self and new experience are relatively compatible, learning is not very disruptive. Bion reminds us, however, that growth is not always characterized by the incremental buildup of manageable experience. Learning can involve intense experiences of emotional turbulence in which meaninglessness can prevail (Billow, 1986). In these instances where the continuous identity (the container) is disrupted by powerfully charged emotional experiences of new knowledge or self-discovery, psychic change can be experienced as catastrophic. Britton (1992) points out that when this happens, the subjective experience is one of fragmentation, inevitably leading to powerful defensive operations involving splitting and projective identification.

If we apply this to the group situation, when powerful thoughts and feelings emerge within the individual that cannot be contained by the person's own containment capacity, they are projected into the group where they may or may not be contained. If these psychic elements cannot be contained within the group, they may threaten to disintegrate the group structure. In other instances, the disruptive psychic elements and the resulting interpersonal turbulence may be exported to the larger system, such as the psychiatric ward where the group takes place. At this juncture the staff and/or patients on the ward may provide a containing function, or the turbulence may move in waves of expansion to the hospital administration, and so on.

In considering the threat of catastrophic change, three factors appear relevant in relation to the outcome of the process evoked by the emergence of new psychic material:

- The power of the disturbing discovery (i.e., the emerging thoughts or feelings)
- The capacity of the container to hold the resulting turbulence (Ps)
- The ability of the container to discover a selected fact, that is, an idea or image that gives coherence to the experience

It is important to remember that groups evolve over time, developing a growing capacity to contain disruptive experience. Groups are, therefore, most vulnerable to the destructive aspects of catastrophic change in their early stages and during transitional phases (e.g., when new members are brought in).

What follows are two clinical vignettes. The first vignette is from a relatively new group. The second vignette is from an established group.

Vignette 1

In an early session of a newly formed therapy group, a 30-year-old male patient told the group that when he was 12 years old, his parents moved from a city where he had lots of friends to a rural area where he was completely isolated. He took a job that summer, working for a well-respected man in the community. It turned out that the man was a pedophile who, over the course of the summer, masturbated the patient on several occasions. The patient said that he really didn't want to talk about this now. He only wanted to mention it, and he felt that these earlier experiences hadn't really affected his adult life.

In a fraction of a second chaos erupted. An older woman who, in her individual therapy, was just beginning to remember sexually inappropriate behavior on the part of both her father and grandfather, exploded with rage, saying, "Well, I think you better look at it. After all, you went over there every day and let him jerk you off." Another woman who was also sexually abused as a child added, "What the hell are you bringing this up for if you don't want to talk about it? If you are not going to talk about your problems, maybe you should leave the group." A male patient started yelling at the two women in defense of the patient who made the disclosure. Another woman said that she thought that people in the group were too hostile and that she was going to leave. A third male said that he was leaving with her, and this all took place in a matter of minutes.

We can see that this early disclosure of powerfully affect-laden material violently shifted the group into a paranoid-schizoid level of organization.

The therapist experienced strong feelings of insecurity, anxiety, confusion, and disorganization, with a sense of dread that the group was on the verge of disintegration. At the height of his intense internal chaos, an intuitive awareness of the group's here-and-now dilemma spontaneously gained coherence in his mind. He told the group that he felt that the patient was right in not wanting to talk about this now. He went on to say, "These experiences are very complicated, powerful and raise anxiety in everyone in here. We will need to deal with them in a thoughtful, sensitive, and understanding way after we get to know each other and trust each other. Our work now is to talk about our feelings about being in this group and maybe some feelings about whether you can trust me and each other not to take advantage of people's loneliness and vulnerability."

The above intervention enabled the group to shift back into a depressive level of organization. The members began to talk about their fears of being in the group and the anxiety related to looking at painful and frightening issues in their lives.

Discussion of Vignette 1

The above vignette emphasizes the fact that the containment process can be much more challenging in the group situations than in dyadic therapy. In the individual therapy situation, the therapist has to worry about her own capacity to contain the projections of her patient. In the group situation, especially in its early life, the group is frequently a poor container, if not a negative container. If we apply Bion's concepts to the vignette just discussed, we can see that the male patient making the premature disclosure was attempting to split off powerful feelings about having been sexually abused. He did this by providing a detailed description of his childhood victimization, while exhibiting little affect and denying the significance of these events. His split-off feelings, especially his disowned rage, were projected into other group members. These feelings, however, could not be contained because the material was too anxiety provoking for at least two of the other members, threatening catastrophic change. The patient who brought the threatening material into the group became the target of a negative containment process, where not only were his own projections returned to him but, in addition, he became the recipient of the other members' rage and anxiety. This shifted the group from what had been a thoughtful, reflective discussion (depressive state of organization) into a paranoid-schizoid state of organization in which there was no tolerance for the various thoughts, images, and feelings that were activated in the group members by the premature disclosure. Some members attempted to make the disclosing patient the repository for all of the group's anxiety and rage. Thoughts were also moving toward actions as members suggested to this particular patient that he should leave the group. Other members threatened to take flight themselves. Fortunately, the therapist's level of internal organization shifted back to a depressive state of organization as a result of an intuitive awareness (selected fact) of the here-and-now issues concerning safety and trust in the early stage of group development. The therapist's intervention served as a container enabling the group members to reintegrate themselves and resume working in a collaborative fashion.

What could have been a containing process around the issue of sexual abuse would have been for the other members of the group to take in the feelings that were split off by the patient who had been sexually abused and be able to bear their own pain and rage long enough to be able to reflect upon it. Eventually each could share their own experiences in an empathic and collaborative way. This did occur over time in the group, and the patient eventually confronted his abuser, seeking and obtaining an apology and financial reparation.

Vignette 2

This second vignette is taken from a group that had been meeting for 2 years. The members had been dealing with issues of intimacy and sexuality.

At the beginning of the session, the therapist announced that a new member would be entering the group in 3 weeks. Although this was followed by the sharing of some fantasies about the new member, the topic was dropped quickly. Ms. A, an attractive 30-year-old, told the group that she had started seeing the group therapist individually because she had developed sexual problems. She thought that she had a lot of guilt about sex, and reported a dream in which she and her boyfriend were at a family picnic. In the dream, the patient and her boyfriend fell into a lake and dirtied it.

A gay male patient in the group, Mr. X, then talked about feeling rejected as a lover by a male friend named Larry, who happened to be a psychiatrist. The patient then added that actually Larry had really wanted the patient, but he rejected Larry on two occasions. Now, Larry, the psychiatrist, likes a mutual friend better. At this point, Ms. B, a somewhat overweight woman, started talking about a friend of hers who recently began to date her old boyfriend. She had set up to have lunch with her female friend, but the friend forgot all about the lunch. The patient was angry but also relieved, because she has a great deal of anxiety about discussing her friend's relationship with her ex-boyfriend.

At this point, Ms. A said, "It seems like we avoided talking about our feelings about the new member." Ms. B said that she hopes that the new member is heterosexual. Then turning to Mr. X, the gay patient, she said, "No offense but I feel that I need feedback from heterosexual men. They are different from you because your friends and sex objects are the same. Like when you were talking about Mo, Larry, and Curly or whoever. It seems like all your friends have been lovers."

Ms. A then said to Ms. B that she felt that "Mr. X should be offended by what you said about his friends, calling them the names of the Three Stooges. It was very demeaning." Ms. B replied that she just has difficulty relating to Mr. X's lovers being his friends. Ms. A then said, "Well, I have a lot of male friends who were once lovers." This hit on Ms. B's sore point. She has had very few men in her life either as lovers or friends.

Ms. B then went off, saying that she did have negative feelings about homosexuals. In fact, she sees them as "frivolous, immoral, and reprehensible." She added that she thinks "it is disgusting and wrong for men to parade around in public in bikini shorts, go to bathhouses, and have 500 or 1,000 sexual contacts. She added that she would feel the same way about women (like Ms. A) who wear short shorts and prance around.

At this point time was up.

Now, while the therapist had had a significant amount of anxiety in the group that was presented in the first vignette, he had confidence that this group of 2 years could come back and work with the potentially explosive and divisive material that was released in this session.

At the beginning of the next session it was reported by Ms. A that in the waiting room, another member, Ms. C, who was absent the previous session, said to Mr. X and Ms. B, "If you two are going to fight, at least wait until I get out of here."

Ms. B then talked about feeling ganged up on last week. She said that she would never bring things up after 8:15 (only a short time remaining in the group). She said that she kept playing the last session over and over in her head all week. She said that she was afraid to come to tonight's session and almost didn't come.

Mr. X said that he was hurt and angry and that he also felt that Ms. B's statements were bigoted. Ms. B began defending herself, saying that she has difficulty with promiscuity and parading around in bikini shorts and going to bathhouses.

Mr. X (attempting to provide a containment function) then said to Ms. B, who is Jewish, "You must have experienced anti-Semitism, where you feel in your gut that someone expressed some anti-Semitic feelings. Words like *frivolous* and *immoral*—that is how gays get labeled. Then people get this picture in their minds, and then you get discriminated against in jobs and housing. Statements like yours reinforce prejudice, and you didn't even temper it with 'Some of my best friends are gay.'" Ms. B argued back that she is distinguishing between behavior and people. Ms. C accused Ms. B of being defensive and not listening.

At this point, the therapist said, "It is natural to defend ourselves, but what we all need to face is the fact that somewhere within us we all have prejudiced feelings. The hard work is to try and look at these feelings and understand them."

Mr. X talked about coming from an anti-Semitic family. Ms. B then added, "Well, as a matter of fact two of my best friends are lesbian and one is a racist. She used to work in Kmart and was constantly talking about the 'coloreds.'" She then added, "I guess if we substituted 'gay' for 'colored,' I would sound a lot like her." A little later she added, "I have been thinking about my envy: I'm envious that gays and the women in this group, especially Ms. A, have it easy in terms of attracting partners and I can't."

Following this, Mr. X said that his prejudices "come out around little things. Like yesterday there was a Black woman on the subway platform snapping her chewing gum and all I could think was how far away could I get away from that Black woman and the sound of that gum." He then said he didn't know why it bothered him so much.

At this point, the therapist suggested that he just imagine the sound of the gum snapping. The patient did this for a few moments and then said that his mother used to snap her gum. The therapist asked him to stay with the sound of the gum snapping. Mr. X then associated to an incident that happened when he was about 12 years old. His mother was snapping her gum in the car. He kept begging her to stop. Instead she just kept saying, "It really doesn't bother you." Finally, he kicked the car window, cracking the glass, ran out of the car, and threw himself on the road. Other group members then joined in and talked about how furious they had been at their parents for not considering their feelings.

The therapist said at this point that he wondered if some of these feelings may also have something to do with the announcement that he was bringing a new member into the group. One member said that she felt that they, the patients, were not considered at all when the therapist decided to bring someone new into the group. Others said they felt angry at the therapist for bringing in a new member at a time when they were feeling particularly close to one another. A member who had come for an individual session imagined that the therapist had a special relationship with the new patient. Another felt that he would not be cared for because new patients get all of the attention.

Toward the end of the group, members began to talk about how they were feeling about each other. Ms. B said to Mr. X, "What really bothered me was that I feel really close to you and the other members in the group, and last week that feeling got threatened." The group ended with a feeling of solidarity related to having been through something together that was trying but important and real.

Discussion of Vignette 2 and Conclusion

The above vignette offers rich material regarding the dynamics of the group and the psychodynamics of the individual patients. The purpose of this paper, however, is more limited and modest: to discuss the relationship between the container, the contained, and the threat of catastrophic change.

In each of the two vignettes, powerful interpersonal and intrapsychic issues (the contained) were activated by the group experience. In the first vignette, the group was in its early stage of development. The patients had not formed cohesive bonds with each other and the therapist. The group, as a container, was relatively undeveloped. The second vignette was taken from an established group that had been meeting for over 2 years. Relationship bonds within the group were strong. The working through of interpersonal conflicts and confrontations was part of the group's history. Although the feelings aroused in this group were as powerful and potentially as divisive as in the first group, the therapist, using himself as a barometer of the threat to the group's integrity, felt a much greater sense of security and confidence that the group could work through the dilemmas it faced. He felt that the group had a strong, vital container that would enable the members to work through the turbulent emotions that had surfaced. Members did, in fact, show themselves to be able to bear and stay with the powerful emotions and process projections in a way that promoted insight and growth. The good object bonds did ultimately triumph over the painful destructive forces of envy, jealousy, shame, fear, and loss.

But what can we expect tomorrow? Careful patient selection, good preparation, and attention to boundaries are absolutely essential to the development of the group as a vital container. Yet we must respect the powerful forces that we are liberating. Serious learning has its inherent risks. Meaningful discovery may require us to bear repeated and endless internal disruptions. The threat of catastrophic change is always there. The group experience threatens our defensive postures and our restrictive self-definitions. It both disorganizes us and helps to rebuild us. But with the risks there is the potential for true discovery as we uncover illusions within ourselves about ourselves. This experience may not always be pleasant, but as Erich Fromm (1960) put it,

> A person senses for the first time that he is vain, that he is frightened, that he hates, while consciously he believed himself to be modest, brave and loving. The new insight may hurt him, but it opens a door; it permits him to stop projecting on others what he represses in himself. He proceeds; he experiences the infant, the child, the adolescent, the criminal, the insane, the saint, the artist, the male and the female within himself; he gets more deeply in touch with his humanity, with the universal man; he represses less and is freer. (pp. 138–139)

References

Billow, R. M. (1986). Bionian interpretation of the Wechsler scales: Paranoid-schizoid operations. In M. Kissen (Ed.), *Assessing object relations phenomena* (pp. 225–267). Madison, CT: Interns. International Universities Press.

Bion, W. R. (1961). *Experiences in groups.* New York: Basic Books.

Bion, W. R. (1962). *Learning from experience.* New York: Basic Books.

Bion, W. R. (1963). *Elements of psycho-analysis.* New York: Basic Books.

Bion, W. R. (1965). *Transformations: Change from learning to growth.* New York: Basic Books.

Bion, W. R. (1967). *Second thoughts: Selected papers on psycho-analysis.* New York: Basic Books.

Bion, W. R. (1970). *Attention and interpretation: A scientific approach to insight in psycho-analysis and groups.* New York: Basic Books.

Bion, W. R. (1977). *Seven servants: Four works by W. R. Bion.* New York: Jason Aronson.

Britton, R. (1992). Keeping things in mind. In R. Anderson (Ed.), *Clinical lectures on Klein and Bion* (pp. 102–113). New York: Routledge.

Eisold, K. (1985). Recovering Bion's contributions to group analysis. In A. Coleman and M. Geller (Eds.), *Group relations reader II* (pp. 37–48). Springfield, VA: Goetz Printing.

Fromm, E. (1960). *Zen Buddhism and psychoanalysis.* New York: Harper Brothers.

Grinberg, L. (1985). Bion's contribution to the understanding of the individual and the group. In M. Pines (Ed.), *Bion and group psychotherapy* (pp. 176–191). London: Routledge & Kegan Paul.

Grinberg, L., Sor, D., & Tabak de Bianchedi, E. (1977). *Introduction to the work of Bion.* New York: Jason Aronson.

James, D. C. (1981). W. R. Bion's contribution to the field of group therapy: An appreciation. In L. R. Wolberg & M. L. Aronson (Eds.), *Group and family therapy* (pp. 28–37). New York: Brunner/Mazel.

James, D. C. (1984). Bion's "containing" and Winnicott's "holding" in the context of the group matrix. *International Journal of Group Psychotherapy, 34*, 201–213.

Klein, M. (1946). Notes on schizoid mechanisms. *International Journal of Psychoanalysis, 27*, 99–110.

Klein, M. (1955). On identification. In M. Klein (Ed.), *Our adult world and other essays.* New York: Basic Books.

Meltzer, D. (1978). *The Kleinian development* (part III). Perthshire: Clunie Press.

Resnik, S. (1985). The space of madness. In M. Pines (Ed.), *Bion and group psychotherapy* (pp 220–246). London: Routledge & Kegan Paul.

Schermer, V. L. (1985). Beyond Bion: The basic assumption states revisited. In M. Pines (Ed.), *Bion and group psychotherapy* (pp. 139–150). London: Routledge & Kegan Paul.

Object Relational and Lacanian Approaches

This section contains papers reflecting the writers' years of development in their writings about basic, universal domains in group therapy.

Dr. Pines brings the authority of his group analytic grasp to bear on the dimension of deep, mutual connection between oneself and other. Placing the subject in the context of culture and history, he turns its many facets to our attention. He writes about the intensity and "sharply exclusive" experience of intimacy as a feature of emotional life, and of definitions of it. Intimacy needs certain recognitions of self and the other to experience it in safety. Among these are communications that make it safe. A group can experience a "we-ness" or "us-ness." Group therapy confronts both the possibility and the risks of the particular safety needed. As group members develop their ties, they continually test whether fellow members imbue their reactions to them and others with sympathetic concern, and even empathy, that they can not only trust but also learn from as models for action and learn about themselves. These judgments are made against their projected fears of being dismissed and depreciated. The more this cable of connectedness, with elements twisting around each other, grows, the more they and others in the group benefit. Nothing can take the place of this absolutely basic and essential experiential learning.

It might seem on first glance at Dr. Pines's title for his second paper is more about systems than individuals' object relations. But here Dr. Pines discusses the group as a container for each individual's dynamics.

Dr. Giraldo has gained a national and international reputation applying concepts from Lacanian theory to psychoanalytic group psychotherapy. Here we have a chance to familiarize ourselves with the ways that he uniquely weaves Lacan's views of the hidden self, of the world of desire and imagination, and of the symbolic order, into the life of a group. Lacan is famously aphoristic and dense. Dr. Giraldo makes him more accessible here.

Other recent references a reader might want to pursue Lacan are the following:

Caudill, D. S. (2000). Lacan's social psychoanalysis: Religion and community in a pluralistic society. In K. R. Malone & S. R. Friedlander (Eds.), *The subject of Lacan: A Lacanian reader for psychologists* (p. 297). New York: State University of New York Press.

Laurent, E. (2000, Spring). The real and the group. *Psychoanalytical Notebooks of the London Circle*, 4, 35.

Barlow, S. H., Taylor, S. M., & Giraldo, M. (2005). Section V: Powerful therapist reactions. In L. Motherwell & J. J. Shay (Eds.), *Complex dilemmas in group therapy: Pathways to resolution*. New York: Brunner-Routledge.

We owe a debt to Dr. Ganzarain for the comprehensive yet succinct way he describes fundamental object relations that create certain particular group processes, and functions of the therapist in dealing with them.

Sy Rubenfeld

Group Analysis and Intimacy

A Whole-Group Approach

Malcolm Pines

The group analytic situation privileges the development of intimate dialogue between persons who are otherwise strangers to each other. Foulkes called this a "proxy" group, where the intimacies of family can be recreated between strangers. The group analytic group however is not only the re-evocation of a family group, for the intimacy and dialogue that can develop between adults transcend the different form of intimacy of a family. The potential for a transformation of character and personality in the group is based on the primary formation of personality and character through the dialogical processes inherent in human life. An understanding and belief in the dialogical principle as constituent of individual life is growing; the relational concepts of psychoanalysis, the increasing understanding of a dialectic or dialogical process of human development all point to the same end. Healthy emotional growth is predicated on the basis of caregiver capacities for emotional attunement, state sharing, turn taking, and play. By these sustained human interactions, healthy infants evolve; in their absence, restricted and impoverished selves develop. Ourselves are given to us to a great extent through the responses of the others, primarily the caregiving couple. It is the Russian philosopher of language Bakhtin who has most clearly enunciated the principle (Holquist, 1990) of "alterity," the other who gives us to ourselves, a concept that can be linked with the Lacanian concept of the other within us. Though Bakhtin's (Clark & Holquist, 1984) writings concentrate on verbal interactions, we can regard nonverbal interactions between infants and caregivers from the start of life as "proto-conversations" (Fogel, 1993) that will gradually become sonorous and later articulate. Though psychoanalysis has in many ways concentrated upon orality as a primary stage in development, this has to be supplemented and in many ways replaced by the significance of the other senses, those of sight and of sound. Human infants are born into a soundbath and the earliest psychic envelope, to use Anzieu's term, is that of the sound envelope. The child is reached to by the intonations of caregivers and its own sounds evoke the sound responses of the caregivers and are intermingled in these earliest forms of intimacy. Soon vision and gaze interaction become salient and we know those moments of rapt intimacy occasioned by the nursing mother seeing for the first time her infant's gaze of recognition as the infant both drinks at the breast and drinks in mother's face through the eyes. I shall quote here from Ralph Waldo Emerson:

> The glance is natural magic. The mysterious communication established across a house between two entire strangers, moves all the springs of wonder. We look into the eyes to know if this other form is another self, and the eyes will not lie, but make a faithful confession what inhabitant is there. The eyes of men converse as much as their tongues, with the advantage that the ocular dialect needs no dictionary but is understood the world over. When the eyes say one thing, and the tongue another, a practiced man relies on the language of the first. If the man is off his centre, the eyes show it. (1860)

It is one of the great distinctions between psychoanalysis and group analysis that the group is a circle of vision, the intercourse of eyes as well as of words.

The dialogical principle has been put forward with great strength by Martin Buber who considers man unique for his ability to be in dialogue with his fellows. The basic fact of human existence is the true dialogue between man and man, based on recognition of the "I" in the otherness of the other and on the readiness of the "I" to listen and respond to the other. In monologue the "I" enables the other to exist only as content of his experience. Buber writes of the realm of the "between," the horizontal depth that group analysis has explored as complement to the vertical depth of psychoanalysis, which explores the individual in the particular social context of the psychoanalytic dyad. In the realm of the "between" people face each other, where they can learn to listen and to accept the other in their entirety, an unfolding of the dialogical. This can be reached in group analysis but only after having overcome many difficulties and it is a process that unfolds haltingly over time. You will recall Buber's famous distinction between the "I-it" relationship and the "I" relationship. I-it relations are partial, essential for many aspects of civilized life but insufficient for nourishing human existence.

In the group there can develop an "us-ness," a "we-ness," in which the group members transcend the boundaries of their own individualities. This is fostered by the nature of the group situation and by the recognition, fostered by the group conductor, of their underlying commonalities both of human existence and of the current group situation.

In the literature on group development, there is an emphasis on pee stages that can be identified and which can lead to the stage of intimacy. But rather than restricting intimacy to a stage of group development I suggest that it is a potentiality that is present in all stages of group life. The development of intimacy cannot be seen as standing apart from those other phenomena of group life, development of capacities for tact, sensitivity, empathy, reciprocity, exchange. The familiar defense mechanisms of repression, denial, projection, and introjection are all constantly at work in the group, yet an understanding of the group process necessitates us going beyond these individualistic notions. In the group we can become intimate with ourselves through the intimacy with others as others give back to us a recognition of those aspects of ourselves that we have either lost or have never recognized.

Intimacy in Group Psychotherapy

In sequential models where phase follows on phase the stage of intimacy is arrived at having passed through the earlier phases. In cyclical models issues to do with intimacy constantly recur as the group moves toward and away from the anxieties that are postulated to underlie existence in the group. In spiral models the issues of intimacy are met again and again at different levels of individual and group capacity or incapacity to cope with the threat and promise of further intimacy (Kron & Youngman, 1987). What then are the fears and promise of intimacy? What can the losses to the individual of a heightening of the quality of intimacy? Intimacy and autonomy are often seen both by patients and by theorists as antagonists; autonomy, the preservation of the self as the center of its own initiative and locus of control, the source of pride and self-esteem, can experience intimacy as a potential plunderer. Fears—of loss of control, of power over oneself, and of being taken over by others more dominant than oneself—will pull the person back within the fortress self. Fears of being pulled back into smothering relationships, being invaded, intruded upon forcefully or insensitively reactivate the fears of early developmental phases; Erikson's basic trust and mistrust. This is the oral phase but in the group this is also connected with aurality, the words of coercion, misattunement, misjudgment. Developing intimacy means entering into more open relationships, a partial handing over power to others, their hope that through this enlargement of oneself, through this more open relationship with the other or others, there will be the rewards of care, solicitude, sympathy, empathy. But intimacy is Janus-faced: There are the risks of rejection, humiliation through wanting from the other what the other is either unwilling or unable to give (Levinger & Raush, 1977). Having entered into an intersubjective phase, being a subject who hopes or expects for the other also to reveal himself as subject, one can suddenly be treated only as an object who is evaluated, criticized, or appraised by another who does not open themselves as another experiencing subject. In developmental terms we can look at this in terms of the state of sharing and the extension of the power of the other to form what Emde calls the "executive we," that gives the sense of "us-ness," two together facing the world as one. Another threat is that by opening oneself to oneself and to others what will be revealed is the "rotten core" that each dreads is uniquely their own before they discover the universality of these negative self-images.

What are the forces driving toward intimacy? There is a sense that this is legitimate, right, and proper in human existence not to live one's life out within the iron cage, the limited horizon of restricted individuality so characteristic of modern societies. Through opening oneself to others there is the possibility of renewal of a sense of vitality, a deeper possibility of self understanding through understanding and internalizing the perspectives of others, of regaining some basic trust and a sense of communion with the world, the communion of early life when we live more subjectively than objectively, as an object both to ourselves and to the scrutiny, surveyance, and control of others (Giddens, 1992).

Levine (1979) writes sensitively and fully about what he calls "Intimacy crises," recurrent phases in group life when the members and the group as a whole hesitate on their stumbling path toward greater intimacy. Withdrawal can take the form of a pseudo-intimacy, Whittaker and Lieberman's restricted solution, a sharing of what all have in common and a refusal to face further differentiation; it can be the deadness of group life, hostility and mistrust, scapegoating or pairing where the intimacy is projected into an individual or a couple to be idealized or forced into acting out forbidden intimacies for the other members. If the therapist is sufficiently aware of these crises and sufficiently comfortable with the idea of group intimacies and of his own partial inclusion and partial exclusion from such intimacies, he can help the group through these crises. What then can develop is a safer sense of inclusion and of autonomy within the group entity, a recognition that intimacy is not a plunderer of autonomy, but its ally. This can be understood in terms of Kohut's self object relationship where the powers of the more developed other are available to the less developed one, the caregiver child relationship, and to Vigotsky's law of proximal development, that the functioning of any one individual cannot be assessed in isolation but only when they are in the presence of a friendly or more knowledgeable other. This is what the group entity itself can become, the more knowledgeable and friendly other, a matrix for development. Then the group entity combines both maternal and paternal functions, the nourishment and containment of the maternal environment together with its stimulation through object presenting, object sharing and play, and the paternal functions of supporting challenge and friendly antagonism (Ross, 1994). The progressive sense of the group as a whole as a helping entity, one that gives a sense of inclusion and autonomy to all its members, that cherishes diversity and individuality, that releases the group from fears of the dominance-submission hierarchy, frees energy for the work of the group, the expression and exploration of both the here and now and the there and then. Foulkes often used the word fellow—a sense of the group members sharing in a community that has a substantial degree of equality and commonality, brotherhood and sisterhood. These terms emphasize the dimension of "the in-between," the horizontal depth, the exploration of what goes on between people that differs significantly from the dyadic relationship where the in-between is only between the members of the dyad, who by the very nature of the dyadic situation are in unequal positions as regard power, knowledge, openness, and responsiveness.

What of conflict? Conflict is always with us but when the group entity assures its members of their acceptance, their being equal members of a common enterprise, then conflicts are less defensive and more productive. Members are free to use their intuitive responses, their deep knowledge of others, the sense of being now an integral part of the lives of each other to respond to the issues that the members bring to the group from the world without and link it with the world within which is the only place of which the members have an authentic basis for knowledge.

Barriers to Intimacy

There are projected fears, the dread of repeating painful existing and earlier experiences, the group transferences (Ormont, 1988); the need to rid the self of feared and loathed parts and to locate them without, the level of the part object transference relationships, the need to act as a receptacle for those projected parts of others that will maintain oneself in the position of the isolate; and there are all the derivatives of shame. I have already dealt with some of the anxieties that derive from the universal human capacity for shame. To be treated as an object by others when one wishes to be treated as a subject to be criticized, humiliated, neglected, excluded. However we must take into account the positive and adaptive qualities of shame, the protector of modesty and from hasty self-exposure to a potentially critical and rejecting world. Modesty brings about the postponement of self-exposure, situations where such actions are likely to be unresponded to with fellow feelings, outside of fellowships that can only be derived from lengthy connection; in close and reciprocal relationships where deeper opening of selves to selves is embedded in the group matrix. Here the sense of shame is adaptive, postponing further opening of the self to others until the right moment, the "kairos," the time outside of chronological time, the propitious moment, the time of revelation, wonder and terrible beauty. We must never neglect the aesthetic dimension of group analysis, the creative response that transforms ugliness into beauty, terror into courage, self-loathing into self-regard.

Broucek (1991) writes, "The sense of shame prevents the libidinal component of the sexual drive from leading us into closer intimacy with another than is compatible with our emotional readiness for such an encounter. When a sense of shame is overridden, and sexual contact with the other is made regardless of our readiness, the situation becomes an analogue of the oral disgust situation and the same affect is apt to be aroused, resulting in disgust toward the objectified other and oneself. The group has to resist the drive toward the sexual relationship and to preserve the erotic dimension, which allows persons to face each other in their rendered identities, aware of their bodily experiences and of the vital dimensions of the sexual. There can be moments of great intimacy when the group gives the opportunity and fosters the capacity for the erotic, for an awareness and enjoyment of the complex and fascinating dimension of human sexual life."

My first published paper (Pines, 1968) was a review of Masters and Johnson, with their description of laboratory sex, sex divorced from intimacy and from the erotic relationship. The sexual arousal of the scientists in viewing their copulating and masturbating subjects had to be suppressed and denied and a "pseudo-objectification" was necessary. Is it a coincidence that their work coincides with the emergence of the encounter movement, of groups where instant and pseudo-intimacy is urged upon the participants? The heady excitements and stimulations of these short-term intimacies, rewarding though they be to some, can often induce an addiction-like state tempting isolated and emotionally impoverished individuals to seek out solutions that are short-term and do not basically alter the underlying pathologies. The slowly developing intimacies of the group analytic situation do offer a sounder solution to our common underlying sense of neurotic overindependence and isolation. I will remind you here of Foulkes's basic thesis that symptoms, inarticulate and autistic, mumbling whilst hoping to be overheard, can in the group situation be articulated, be exchanged for language that communicates responsively with others, where the barriers to intimacy gradually dissolve, where through fellowship the self can be replenished, be reaffirmed, and reemerge more able to deal with ongoing developmental tasks and opportunities of individual life (de Swaan, 1990).

References

Broucek, F. J. (1991). *Shame and the self.* New York: Guilford Press.

Clark, K., & Holquist, M. (1984). *Mikhail Bakhtin.* Cambridge: Harvard University Press.

Emerson, R. W. (1860). Behavior. In *The conduct of life.*

Fogel, A. (1993). *Developing through relationships: Origins of communication, self and culture.* Chicago: University of Chicago Press.

Giddens, A. (1992). *The transformation of intimacy: Sexuality, love and eroticism in modern societies.* Cambridge: Polity Press.

Holquist, M. (1990). *Dialogist: Bakhtin and his world.* London: Routledge.

Kron, T., & Youngman, R. (1987). The dynamics of intimacy in group therapy. *International Journal of Group Psychotherapy, 37,* 529–548.

Levine, B. (1979). *Group psychotherapy: Practice and development.* Englewood Cliffs: Prentice Hall.

Levinger, G., & Raush, H. L. (Eds.). (1977). *Close relationships: Perspectives on the meaning of intimacy.* Amherst: University of Massachusetts Press.

Ormont, L. (1988). The leader's role in resolving resistances to intimacy in the group setting. *International Journal of Group Psychotherapy, 38,* 29–45.

Ross, J. M. (1994). *What men want: Motherhood, fatherhood and manhood.* Cambridge: Harvard University Press.

Swaan, A. de. (1990). *The management of normality.* London: Routledge.

The Group-as-a-Whole Approach in Foulkesian Group Analytic Psychotherapy

MALCOLM PINES

The distinctive feature that marks group analysis out from other schools of group psychotherapy—and from psychoanalysis—is the firmly held basic assumption that the distinctions that are usually made between "individual" and "group" are unnecessary and artificial. The precious notion that we all cling to our own individuality and ownership of our own minds—"I am master of my body and captain of my soul" (N. Pines, 1925 onward!) as the 19th century attempted to proclaim—is indeed but a notion or theory. Foulkes asserted that the real nature of what we call "mind" arises from each individual's need for communication and for reception. Language goes on in the mind of the individual and is experienced as one's own thoughts, but language is a shared property of the group and originates in our needs for communication, for survival and adaptation (Foulkes & Anthony, 1957, p. 244). This means that the individual is penetrated to the very core by culture and grows into "normality" quite unconscious of those colossal social forces that have shaped and molded him or her. The full nature of an individual's psychic reality can only be seen by situating the person in context, on the ground from which they originate. Here we see Foulkes's indebtedness to Kurt Goldstein, the psychologist and neurologist, with whom he had worked and who so strongly emphasized the figure-ground concept for the functioning of the organism. Beyond the infantile amnesia and defenses that protect this unconscious repression, above and beyond this, we are unaware, ignorant of much of our psychic makeup, of our cultural attitudes, not because they are repressed but because we are convinced that they are right and proper and need not be examined. The restricted range of what we term "normality" is made clear to us when we are in contact with other cultures, looking glasses to some of the most basic of human physical and mental functions. We take for granted how we cat, excrete, exchange, and fashion the business of our daily lives. Thrown into other contexts than our own, other sounds, languages, positions, affiliations, we discover that our sense of safety and wholeness is to a large part based on being part of a socio-psychological network.

Network

This concept of "network" is at the basis of group-analytic theory. Foulkes defined an individual as a person occupying a nodal place in the social network, again deriving this concept from the Gestalt psychology of Kurt Goldstein (Goldstein, 1939; Foulkes, 1990, pp. 39–56). Goldstein, a profound philosopher of biology, had studied the response of the injured, brain-damaged person and had demonstrated that it is the whole person who actively responds to and attempts to adapt to injury of the central nervous system. In disease, the equilibrium of the central nervous system cannot be maintained, and the damaged part, instead of functioning as a nodal point in the network, now represents a focal point for disequilibrium to which the whole organism now has to adapt. By analogy, there is a social network, which forms and in many ways "is" the person, and in illness we can trace processes of disturbance in the network, which then manifest through one person, the presenting patient, as "illness." These processes are very clear in infant and child psychiatry and can be revealed in the world of adults, provided that we are prepared to examine and to understand the sociopsychological background. This approach is well supported by research—for instance, the studies of the relationship of depression in women to particular social processes (Brown & Harris, 1978).

Some assert that the group-analytic approach is mainly socio-psychological, which replaces the psychoanalytic depth of study of the individual by a more superficial study of group life, but this is an inaccurate attribution and categorization Foulkes repeatedly stated that the "social" is deeply inside each one of us, and what seems to be "outside" or "inside" is itself a construct by ourselves and by our cultures. Individual and social, intra- and interpersonal, are, like the Möbius strip, eternally unfolding and unfolding. This is what the group-analytic situation enables each one of us to recognize and experience. It is in this group-analytical experience that we can begin to appreciate the degree to which we are bound together through unconscious forces. As Foulkes wrote, "The very fact that we can easily understand each other and that this understanding can extend to such depth, is a token of our membership of a shared culture" to which he gave the name of "foundation matrix" (Foulkes, 1990, pp. 223–233).

The Group-as-a-Whole

The concept of group-as-a-whole is intrinsic to group analysis; it was there from the start. Foulkes wrote the following in his first book:

While having an eye on each individual member and on the effects they and their utterances have on each other, the conductor is always observing and treating the group-as-a-whole. The group-as-a-whole is not a phrase; it is a living organism, as distinct from the individuals, composing it. It has moods and reactions, a spirit, an atmosphere, a climate. . . . One can judge the prevailing climate by asking oneself: "What sort of thing could or could not possibly happen in this group? What could be voiced?" (1948: 140) The conductor can gauge his own distance to the group by asking himself, "What sort of thing could I say within this situation, and what could not be said?" In fact, it is the group-as-a-whole with which the conductor is primarily in touch and he experiences its individuals inside the setting. You should sense what this group needs at any given moment, be it encouragement, reassurance, or stimulation, steadying or excitation. (Foulkes, 1948, p. 140)

Foulkes's capacity to grasp this notion and to base both theory and practice on it arose from his recognition of the depth and strength of social forces in the human psyche. For him society is not "outside" the person: it is internal and penetrates to the innermost being of the individual. Thus within a given culture persons are rooted together in a foundation matrix, sharing not only a common language but also unconsciously holding common assumptions regarding the most basic of life processes—feeding, excreting, and sleeping, and assumptions as to the nature of their world. Undoubtedly he had understood this from the seminal work of the sociologist colleague whom he had met in Frankfurt, Norbert Elias, whose book *The Civilizing Process* Foulkes had introduced to the psychoanalytic world in 1936 (Foulkes, 1948; Mennell, 1989).

Thus Foulkes's concept of working with a small group did not represent an individualistic psychoanalytic position, whereby a therapist can observe and treat numbers of patients instead of one at a time, an economy of time. From the start he regarded the group as an entity in itself, a "common matrix within which all relationships develop" and "axiomatic that everything happening in a group involves the group-as-a-whole as well as each individual member" (Foulkes, 1949, p. 49).

By firmly holding on to this concept the group analyst can consider the ways in which individuals take part in the therapeutic process, which also enables the therapist to intervene at an individual level when this seems appropriate. This gives the therapist a degree of freedom of action that may not be allowed to one who needs to confine his or her actions solely to the group-as-a-whole level.

At this point I shall briefly consider how other persons have used the group-as-a-whole concept, as there is much confusion on this issue that I hope to clarify.

W. R. Bion (Pines 1985)

The approach initiated by Bion is well known to predicate unconscious modes of functioning of the group in relation to its leader and to its work task. Powerful and primitive forces acting as resistances to the work of therapy hold the group in thrall. These patterns that Bion termed "basic assumptions" are those of dependency, fight-flight, and pairing. His assumption was that interpretation of these patterns could release the blocked work capacity and that this was the major, indeed the prime, task of the group therapist. Though Bion recognized that man is a group creature who is at war with his social nature, he did not elaborate on the rootedness of humans in their social structure, in contrast to Foulkes. This leads to a considerable limitation in applying his ideas to group life in general.

The same argument applies to Henry Ezriel (Ezriel, 1973), who based his work on a schema of how object relations would reappear in the group setting. His work represents the strict application of one version of psychoanalytic theory to the group setting and fails to take into account the intrinsic dynamics of group life or indeed the fundamental sociality of human life.

Dorothy Stock Whitaker (Whitaker 1985)

A far more flexible and illuminating scheme is set out by this author. Her work was considerably influenced by Bion through his concept of group mentality but, since then, has gone on independently and with originality. Less influenced by psychoanalytic theory, though acknowledging the work of Thomas French on "focal conflict," she has integrated many aspects of social psychology and group dynamics in her important writings. On the whole, her work is more concerned with "nonclinical" settings, studying how group dynamics appear in all group situations. She studies how group themes emerge through the flow of associations, how norms and belief systems develop in the course of group life, and what solutions they offer to the inevitable dilemmas of individuals interacting in groups. She writes that the "group as a whole can be described in terms of mood or atmosphere, shared schemes, norms and belief systems, structure, boundaries, roles and role distinctions, conflict, consensus and developmental stages," and writes that "whole group phenomena are generated by the interaction of group members but they are not merely the sum of individual contributions. They can properly be said to 'belong' to the group as a whole."

Dorothy Whitaker's comprehensive and well-argued theory is a powerful and useful tool for therapists. Where Foulkes differs is again in his insistence on the power of those social and cultural forces within the individual that go into the formation of both normal personality and of its disorders. His concepts of network, matrix, and group-specific forces are distinctive. But the group analyst can learn much from Dorothy Whitaker's technique, but needs also to retain the more psychoanalytic nature of observing without intervening until she or he feels the need to do so. This need may lead to interaction with individuals as well as with the group-as-a-whole and will not necessarily deal with the developmental conflicts of group life that Dorothy Whitaker has so well illuminated.

Yvonne Agazarian

In Agazarian's group-as-a-whole theories and also possibly in her practice there are considerable resemblances to Dorothy Whitaker. This is not surprising, as they both declare an allegiance to Lewin's social psychology and to the group dynamic researches that were stimulated by him from the 1950s onwards. But Agazarian has pioneered a group-as-a-whole approach that applies systems theory systematically and most definitely gives the group prime place for the observations and actions of the group conductor.

Her theory of the "invisible group" (Agazarian & Peters, 1981) presents group concepts that are distinct and discrete from individual psychology. It is an integrational system theory that spells out the structure and functions of individual and group dynamics as two discrete but related systems. The conductor observes from two perspectives—individual and group systems—that coexist simultaneously in space and time. The individual dynamics are characteristically expressed in member-role behavior, modified by interaction in the group; unconscious group-as-a-whole dynamics are expressed in characteristic group-as-a-whole role behavior that affects the development of the group-as-a-whole and that in turn affects individual group members. Agazarian keenly observes processes of group development and differentiation and takes subgroups as the basic unit of observation, not any one individual. Subgroups make visible the boundaries that are developing, boundaries that contain differences that need to be made visible for the group to pursue the group's developing problem-solving skills (Agazarian, 1989).

Agazarian is constantly further developing her work within the systems framework, and the contribution of psychoanalytic theory plays a lesser part. The conductor's role in Agazarian's work is clearly observable and definable in monitoring and aiding the development of the group as a problem-solving situation. In contrast, the group-analytic therapist's role is not so well defined or described, which allows for the development of individual styles that reflect both the personality and beliefs of the conductor but which, despite many apparent differences, all rest on the same group-analytic theory base.

My own understanding of the group-as-a-whole concept has been developing over a number of years. Working with groups that meet over a very long period of time, either once or twice a week, I have had the opportunity to observe and indeed to wonder at the capacity of group members to create a working unity, a body of persons who share a psychic life within the group boundary of space and time. Even if only meeting once a week they can develop a depth of experience and of understanding of that experience that remarkably changes some aspects of each individual's psychic life. It is clear that this must arise from the transformational potential of the group situation and the fact that the burden of the work is carried by the group members themselves. They engage in exploration and understanding both one another's individual mentalities and, increasingly, the way in which each functions within the group and what is carried for the other as well as for themselves. Gradually, psychic boundaries seem to become more permeable, the boundaries that define each one person as distinct from another—the "self boundary," in a sense—and those boundaries that define the inner structure of each individual. These are the boundaries between conscious and unconscious, internal boundaries of self- and other representations, of the psychic structures of ego, superego, and id, the boundary between reality and fantasy and so on. For many persons, such changes in self-definition make possible the useful interpenetration of one person's mind by another's; for other persons, what is needed is a strengthening of those boundaries so that the person becomes less open to what is experienced as invasion or intrusion.

Thus over time there seems to be an increasing sense of "fitting in" of the group members, creating what to myself as participant observer, and I believe to the group members also, is an increasing sense of coherency. I shall address this issue of coherency later but for now confine the meaning of the word to a sense of understanding what is going on, that it makes sense and becomes increasingly meaningful.

At the start Foulkes borrowed the term "psyche group" from Moreno's colleague Helen Jennings. He gave depth and strength to this concept by introducing his own concept of the group matrix. As this is discussed elsewhere in this volume I will restrict my own comments to the matrix as an evolutionary concept that refers to the developmental history of a group which is based upon the communicational network laid down by its participants over time. On the basis of this communicational network a form of psychological organization develops in a group based upon mutual experiences, relationships, and understandings. The shared history of interpersonal relationships in the group and of the shared work in deriving meaning from their work together lays down this dynamic group matrix. It is this process that establishes a deeper sense of coherency, both conscious and unconscious, that I believe is intrinsic to the concept of the group-as-a-whole.

The Two Meanings of the Word *Group*—
Cohesion and Coherency (Pines, 1986)

I have always been struck by the wisdom of words, and I want to consider our basic word *group* in this respect. According to the *Shorter Oxford English Dictionary* there are two roots for the word *group*; one is Germanic and the other Latin. The more ancient Germanic origin of the word *group* is derived from the word for "crop," that is, the gizzard of a bird. For within the crop of an animal is to be found an agglomeration of substances that have been swallowed and that have lost their discrete nature and are now clumped together to form a fibrous mass. Thus in individual elements partly digested, glued together to form a bolus, we can see the image of a primitive group. This is a group where elements stick together, now partly changed by being mixed—together in this agglomeration that has an external boundary, being shaped now into a sort of ball but that lacks any internal structure. The force that holds this mass together can be termed *cohesion*. My dictionary defines *cohesion* as "unity of material things held together by a physical substance such as cement, mortar, glue or by a physical force such as attraction or affinity." This well describes the sticky mass of the organic bolus but also can be used as a metaphor to describe some aspects of group life. A group that sticks together displays a force that will resist being pulled apart, will resist invasion. In group psychology there has been a great deal of attention paid to this concept of cohesion, and it has been put forward as a cardinal principle for group psychotherapy. Groups that do not hold together, that do not exert a force of attraction or affinity for their members, do not develop the capacity for psychological work, for experiencing and dealing with the psychic work that is involved in facing painful issues. It has also been recognized that the forces of cohesion can act as resistances to differentiation and development, and it is possible to see Bion's basic assumptions, for instance, as instances of powerful group cohesive forces.

The other origin for the word *group* comes from the Latin, and is connected with a concept of "grouping" as an active process. No longer the passive agglomeration of only partly differentiated substances, *grouping* refers to objects that are actively grouped together in order to display an organizational principle. The dictionary defines *coherence* as unity, firstly of immaterial, of intangible things, such as the points of an argument, the details of a picture, the incidents, characters, and setting of a story; or secondly of material and of objective things that are bound into a unity by a spiritual, intellectual, or aesthetic relationship, as through their clear sequence or their harmony with one another. It therefore commonly connotes an integrity that makes the whole and the relationship of its parts clear and manifest. So here we have the dictionary describing "an integrity which makes the whole and the relationship of its parts clear and manifest."

It is this concept of coherency that I wish to put forward as perhaps the prime factor in the evolution of "the group-as-a-whole" (Pines, 1986). The group-analytic group meets under conditions set down and maintained by the group analyst as "dynamic administrator." Thus the basic issues of time, space, reliability, confidentiality, the privilege of verbal communication over action, the understanding that people meet together in order to increase their understanding of themselves and thereby to gain greater mastery over their inner lives are the basis of the work. These organizational principles are part of the group analyst's own mentality, derived from his or her training and position in the training matrix of the group-analytic community. It is this basic structure that will be tested again and again through the life of the group and that gradually becomes internalized by the group members themselves, so that in the long run they themselves become the organizers of the group (Pines, 1985). Thus each member of the group occupies the position of a "double agent," both member and recipient of the group processes but also supporter and vital link in the group structure. Thereby the group members gradually come to work at "higher" levels of psychic organization, maturing over time as the life of the group develops; this double process plays an increasing part in holding the group together and yet at the some time allows members to experience deeper, more regressive, more loosely organized aspects of self through their own inner explorations and through participation in the psychic lives of the other group members.

To return to the developmental aspects of the group matrix, I find it helpful to think about the group in terms of an increasing coherence that makes the whole and the relationship of its parts more clear and manifest. My achievement of coherence in the group process enables its members to retrace the developmental path of coherence in childhood (Pines, 1985). The path of childhood development can be seen as the organism's gradual attainment of a state of coherency; concepts of self and of identity all imply development of a form of coherency, the parts fitting together to make a whole. Now that studies of child development increasingly center on the observation of the mother-infant pair, the concept of coherency again comes to the fore. How do any particular infant-mother or caregiver pairs fit together? How much intuitive or intelligent understanding is displayed by the caregiver towards any one particular child, and what are the capacities of any particular child to respond "understandingly" to the actions of the caregiver? We know that there is a whole range of possibilities between the harmonious interplay of a skilled intuitive caregiver with a responsive and receptive infant, and the painfully destructive incapacity of the pair to relate to each other. Modern observational techniques allow for the recognition of the most subtle example of successful and unsuccessful translation of impulses and needs by the infant and successful or unsuccessful response of the caregiver.

All this can be subsumed under the concept of "dialogue," a process that begins as interplay of gestures that gradually lead on to the precursors of conversations, finally arriving at the stage of verbalizations (Leal, 1982). All the time the infant is being drawn into communication with the social world, internalizing the gestures of the social world that are offered to it and that are also offered as responses to the infant's own gestures. Thus, as Foulkes so clearly saw, the social is laid down deeply within the individual from the very start. For this is a language of gestures that belongs both to the most intensely personal, to the unique mother-caregiver dyad, but also to that set of responses communicated through culture to the caregivers as the appropriate gestures to make to infants.

Within the realm of developmental psychology it is to Vygotsky that we have to turn for a satisfactory model to explain this form of development. Vygotsky spoke of the "law of proximal development" (Weitsch, 1985). By this he meant that the social world, the caregivers, are always drawing the infant onto the next possible stage of development. They are offering gestures to the infant for the infant to grasp, initially by chance but then to build into the infant's own behavioral repertoire, that show an understandable and intelligible response.

Coherence and Narrative

The persons sharing the therapy group under group-analytic conditions (free group discussion, slow/open group with consistent membership over lengthy periods, conductor maintaining a mostly interpretative stance) are basically constructing narratives of current and past life experiences. These narratives will be reshaped through the reception given by their fellow group members. This reshaping virtually gives expression to a new coherency for the persons—a life story that gives fuller weight to development in the context of family, as that context is to some extent replayed in the here and now of the group (see Chapter 6, by Dennis Brown). Thus, for each person, there are two personal narratives, the here and now in the group and there and then, in the past, and it is the dynamic juxtaposition of these stories that gradually fits the two together. Robin Skynner has addressed this in terms of the "templates" that the group members gradually fit together (Skynner, 1986).

Group members mostly enter therapy in the hope of finding relief from suffering without radical change; the search for self-understanding gradually becomes the prime mover, as persons discover that this is predominantly what the situation offers, aid to self-understanding through work with others engaged in the same enterprise. Self-understanding is the search for what unifies our diverse experiences with our fantasies, our dreams, our relations with others.

Coherence and Metaphor

The philosophers Lakoff and Johnson (1980) argue that metaphors are not merely a matter of words, for human thought processes are largely metaphorical. Metaphors bind elements into coherent systems, and if you look at the structure of our language, we express a multitude of experiences through metaphors, many of which are related to the body image. From birth onward, our body image, with the dimensions of vertical, horizontal, and depth, becomes a way of expressing experience. Upness is connected with happiness, health, consciousness, awakeness; downness, with illness, sadness, grossness, the hidden aspects of the self, with the unconscious. Western society privileges the vertical, and psychoanalysis gives persons the opportunity to plunge into the depths of the self. Eastern cultures privilege the horizontal, and emphasize balance and harmony. In a group-analytic situation, the horizontal dimension, the self in relationship to others, has to be acknowledged and worked at, at the same time as each individual can also come into contact with their own vertical depth. Thus, the bringing together of the vertical and the horizontal, the in-between and the within, is part of the coherency that may be achieved by group members.

The Group Setting

Metaphors of holding and containment are increasingly applied to analytic groups. They usefully express the reality of a situation, where persons allow themselves to relate to others at depth. Deeply significant relationships develop that involve powerful affects, and were there not a sense of reliability and strength of the group setting these developments could not take place. As developed by Winnicott and Bion, containing and holding refer to very early relationship experiences (see Chapter 5, by Colin James). Holding is a metaphor based on the physical experience, the holding that caregivers give to infants, but is a metaphor that coherently brings together a great variety of parental, predominantly material, acts and attitudes. Containment relates to the maternal capacity to take in, to understand, and to appropriately respond to an infant's needs, which are predominantly expressed through distress.

By an understanding that leads to an appropriate response, the caregiver creates a coherent pattern out of the infant's initially inchoate actions. The infant seems to begin to understand hunger as part of a relationship in which hunger will be communicated, understood, and responded to by food and by loving care, so that the infant's emotional needs will be fed at the same time as the physiological needs are satisfied. In group analysis, the group-as-a-whole, formed by the members and the conductor together, takes on these functions of holding and containment, so that individual needs are fairly reliably understood and responded to appropriately (Kosseff, 1991).

Within psychoanalytic theory, Hans Loewald addressed this notion of coherency as a major therapeutic process. Freud had described the ego as "a coherent organization of mental processes," many of which are functioning at an unconscious level. Thus, there is a distinction between the coherent unconscious and the repressed unconscious fantasies, which are not organized under this principle of coherency. Regarding the therapeutic process as one in which the patient internalizes aspects of the interaction process between patient and therapist, what is inter- becomes an inherent part of the coherent ego. Thus, there is an exchange between the more primitive, chaotic, and incoherent parts of the unconscious self, largely expressed through responses to the therapeutic situation manifested through the transference. There is an exchange process whereby the primitive is understood and responded to by the therapist, who acts at a higher, more organized level both of consciousness and unconsciousness. The therapist's intuition and countertransference responses arise from the unconscious coherent ego and thus, through internalization processes, the therapist's responses become part of a new organization of the patient's unconscious mental life. Loewald writes:

> It is of the utmost importance, theoretically and clinically, to distinguish more clearly and consistently than Freud ever did between processes of repression and processes of internalization. The latter are involved in creating an increasingly coherent integration and organization of the psyche *as a whole* [my italics], whereas repression works against such

coherent psychic organization, by maintaining a share of psychic processes in a less organized, more primitive state.

As I have written elsewhere:

> There is an essential paradox in the group situation. The basic function of holding and containment coexist with a culture that is based on analysis and translation, which are sophisticated levels of higher functioning. Thus, there are inherent contradictions in the group situation, a delicate, stable, yet unstable balance that has constantly to be monitored and managed. Early developmental processes reenacted in the group can be held, contained, and tolerated as the group can function at a higher level and is available to the individuals, often more adequately and appropriately than were the containers and holders for patients' early experiences. Thus, members develop their capacity to think in the face of pain and to tolerate and to know the unthinkable. (Pines, unpublished)

So, finally, I come to an attempt to define the group-as-a-whole in group-analytic terms: It is the basic concept underlying the approach to a group that meets in a standard group-analytic situation, which privileges communication and in which the therapeutic aim is to enable both individual and group coherency to emerge over time at both conscious and unconscious levels. Increased unconscious coherency represents the establishment and enrichment of the group matrix.

Note: The special issue of the journal *Group* (13: 3–4) is devoted to "the-group-as-a-whole." Edited by Yvonne Agazarian, it contains a comprehensive overview of contemporary approaches to the topic.

References

Agazarian, Y. (1989). Group-as-a-whole systems and practice. *Group, 13*: 1301–1354.
Agazarian, Y., & Peters, R. (1981). *The visible and the invisible group.* London: Routledge & Kegan Paul.
Broucek, F. J. (1991). *Shame and the self.* New York: Guilford Press.
Brown, G. W., & Harris, T. (1978). *Social origins of depression: A study of psychiatric disorders in women.* London: Tavistock.
Clark, K., & Holquist, M. (1984). *Mikhail Bakhtin.* Cambridge: Harvard University Press.
Emerson, R. W. (1860). Behavior. In *The conduct of life.*
Ezriel, H. (1973). Psychoanalytic group theory. In L. R. Wolberg & E. Schwartz (Eds.). *Group Therapy 1973. An overview.* New York: International Medical Books.
Fogel, A. (1993). *Developing through relationships: Origins of communication, self and culture.* Chicago: University of Chicago Press.
Foulkes, S. H. (1948). *Introduction of group-analytic psychotherapy.* London: Mansfield.
_____. (1990). *Selected papers: Psychoanalysis and group analysis* (ed. Elizabeth Foulkes). London: Karnac Books.

_____. (1990). Biology in the light of the work of Kurt Goldstein. In E. Foulkes (Ed.). *Selected papers: Psychoanalysis and group analysis* (chap. 4). London: Karnac Books.

_____. (1990). The group as matrix of the individual's mental life. In E. Foulkes (Ed.). *Selected papers: Psychoanalysis and group analysis* (chap. 22). London: Karnac Books.

Foulkes, S. H., & Anthony, E. J. (1957). *Group psychotherapy: The psycho-analytic approach*. Harmondsworth: Penguin; 2nd ed. 1965. Reprinted 1984 London: Karnac.

Giddens, A. (1992). *The transformation of intimacy: Sexuality, love and eroticism in modern societies*. Cambridge: Polity Press.

Goldstein, K. (1939). *The organism*. New York: American Books.

Holquist, M. (1990). *Dialogist: Bakhtin and his world*. London: Routledge.

Kosseff, J. W. (1991). Infant and mother and the mother–group. In S. Tuttman (Ed.). *Psychoanalytic group theory and therapy* (pp. 133–156). Madison, CT: International Universities Press.

Kron, T., & Youngman, R. (1987). The dynamics of intimacy in group therapy. *International Journal of Group Psychotherapy, 37*, 529–548.

Lakoff, G., & Johnson, M. (1980). *Metaphors we live by*. Chicago: University of Chicago Press.

Leal, R. (1982). Resistances and the group analytic process. *Group Analysis, 15*: 97–110.

Levine, B. (1979). *Group psychotherapy: Practice and development*. Englewood Cliffs: Prentice Hall.

Levinger, G., & Raush, H. L. (Eds.). (1977). *Close relationships: Perspectives on the meaning of intimacy*. Amherst: University of Massachusetts Press.

Loewald, H. W. (1980). *Papers on psycho-analysis*. New Haven, CT: International Universities Press.

Mennell, S. (1989). *Norbert Elias: Civilisation and the human self-image*. Oxford: Blackwell.

Ormont, L. (1988). The leader's role in resolving resistances to intimacy in the group setting. *International Journal of Group Psychotherapy, 38*, 29–45.

Pines, M. (Ed.). (1985). *Bion and group psychotherapy*. London: Routledge & Kegan Paul.

_____. (1985). Psychic development and the group analytic situation. *Group, 9*: 24–37.

_____. (1986). Coherency and its disruption in the development of the self. *British Journal of Psychotherapy, 2*: 180–185.

Ross, J. M. (1994). *What men want: Motherhood, fatherhood and manhood*. Cambridge: Harvard University Press.

Swaan, A. de. (1990). *The management of normality*. London: Routledge.

Weitsch, J. V. (1985). *Vygotsky and the social formation of mind* (p. 67). Cambridge, MA: Harvard University Press.

Winnicott, D. W. (1986). What is effective in group psychotherapy? *Group Analysis, 19*(1): 5–22.

Whitaker, D. W. (1985). *Using groups to help people*. London: Routledge.

Chaos and Desire

The Simple Truth of the Unconscious
in the Psychoanalytic Group

MACARIO GIRALDO

Recently I went for a routine haircut in the suburb where I live. As the haircut proceeded I began to feel drowsy. When I was done I turned to my barber, a short, unassuming young lady. I said to her: "I was so relaxed; I was beginning to fall asleep." To which she responded, very matter-of-factly, "Well, you like to be touched." Her words came upon me as if some curtain had been moved from my eyes. I saw something familiar to me, some simple truth that has since elaborated gradually in my mind, the product, I think, of my past work in analysis. Furthermore, I had a very pleasant feeling. Here was this young woman, very similar in attitude and simplicity to my sisters and the country people I originate from, giving me a message that she could not know told me a lot about myself at that moment. In a sense, I was getting the benefit of a bit of analysis from somebody who, using the curtain of words, of signifiers, as Lacan puts it, removed the blinds to a room of my interior that had been nicely protected by my drowsiness. Here was an aspect of my unconscious, drawn out cleverly by a matter-of-fact interpretation. The lady barber heard my words and responded. Her message surprised me for a moment but led me to the reading of a familiar inscription that she pointed out to me unobtrusively. Something landed in my mind with the weight of a simple truth.

A barbershop is a group room, a place where stories are told and heard. Comments are made that can be at the same time totally frivolous and inspiring, soothing and boring. It is a room where several people come for a similar purpose, yet, each one likes to have their hair done in a special way; a place where each person talks as if he is alone with the barber, yet the room is usually filled with the presence of other customers. A barbershop acts as a group container for individual dialogues that the barber learns to hear as the uninterrupted monologues of his customers. Perhaps, the barbershop is akin to the psychoanalytic group.

Let me move away from this barbershop to my group-room where I practice psychoanalytic group psychotherapy. Most of the time, in this room, I am the designated "barber." But the reality is that in the psychoanalytic group each member is potentially a barber and a customer. I will present to you a situation from a group in transition and will attempt to explore some aspects of the work with the unconscious in the psychoanalytic group.

I had been conducting two therapy groups. The number of patients had come down to five in one group and four in the other. I began to consider inviting these two groups to join in one new group. I had several ideas in mind—to have a better mix of men and women, to facilitate the work with a variety of issues with a richer dynamic in the new group, and to test the patients' disposition and my own to undertake this change which could prove beneficial but also present some difficulties. After some personal struggle as to the pros and cons, I presented my decision to each group and gave them two months to work on the thoughts and feelings related to this change.

One group, Group A, had two women, Arcadia and Julia, and three men, Rodrigo, Alvaro, and Stanford. The other group, Group B, had one man, Jonathan, and three women, Adele, Belinda, and Ortencia. Let me call Group A the optimistic group, and Group B the mixed group.

A central character in Group A was Arcadia. This was her second round of group therapy. In the past her common reaction to any new person entering her group was very negative. In this case she said that she was surprised by her own reaction. She now looked forward to the merger and felt this would add new life to the group. The other members, Julia, Rodrigo, Alvaro, and Stanford, fell somewhere between looking forward to it and a wait-and-see attitude.

In Group B, Adele was a central character. She responded very negatively to the idea and said that she most likely would leave the group. Among many of the reasons that she gave one had to do with Stanford, a member of Group A.

Adele's group knew of Stanford. He had been in her group for a brief period of time and then withdrawn one year before. In making the announcement of the merger I told Adele's group that Stanford had come back into therapy and was now a member of Group A. I felt that this was information that Group B needed to have.

Stanford became for Adele a central representation for her negative reactions. He was a young man in his mid-20s, about half Adele's age. He appeared often as withdrawn, angry, and tense. She felt that she had enough difficulty dealing with men close to her age and that Stanford was way beyond her reach, somebody to whom she could not relate. She could not see herself opening up with him in the group. She remembered an interaction with him before his withdrawal from the group where he had expressed strong negative comments to her.

Adele had been in group psychotherapy previously, with another therapist, and felt that she had benefited a great deal from it. She was then in individual therapy with somebody else but came to a point of feeling stuck and not being able to move forward. She had stopped that therapy and come to me for group and individual therapy. She had been in treatment for two years with me. Adele's basic complaints related to intense feelings of loneliness, doubts about being able to find a man and be married. She had had a number of men in her life but had not been able to meet the one that she could marry. This new effort at therapy was motivated by the failure of an important relationship with a man she was quite fond of. Adele's basic comment on the group merger was: I am not going to change anyway, so it is useless for me to start all over again with a new group. She repeated this theme in a variety of ways during the session prior to the merger.

The first session of the new group was eventful. Rodrigo, who had been absent for five weeks because of job-related travel, was rather abrupt in reacting to a story by Julia about her new church. He used a four-letter word to describe those who go to church. Julia was upset at Rodrigo's flippant comment. Arcadia joined in, and Alvaro felt that Rodrigo was going back to old behavior. So basically all of the members of Group A (my "optimistic group") had a very mixed response to Rodrigo's opening salvo coming from within their own ranks. However, Alvaro was quick to point to Group B that Rodrigo was actually a very soft and warm man, very intelligent and highly cultivated.

In Group B, Belinda was missing because of surgery. Adele went on to list her reasons for not staying in the group. Ortencia was quiet but obviously struck by what was going on in the group and concerned about Adele's continuing threats of leaving. She did not want her to leave the group. She felt very identified with some of her complaints. As for Jonathan, he became almost immobilized by Rodrigo's salvo. He said he did not know what to say, he could not find words. He added, though, that he found his own reaction to Rodrigo's comment quite remarkable. In this first session Group A appeared for a moment rather chaotic and Group B was in shock and with a passive stance toward the newcomers. Let me present other pieces of dialogues from another session within the first month of the merger.

In this session Belinda is still missing because of surgery. Julia announces that she is she is deciding to change careers and move from a highly technical and well-paid computer manager's role to become a high school teacher. I ask Stanford about his thoughts on Rodrigo's comments and he basically growls at me and tells me that he has no thoughts. To this, Rodrigo comments, "Well, the way you answered Dr. Giraldo, it is not as if you have no thoughts." Stanford goes on to tell the group that he was run off the road by a drunken driver the night before. He had to walk for a mile and a half.

Th: Are you glad you are alive?
S.: Yes.
Th.: Some time ago you would not have felt that way.
S.: I think you are right.

This leads to a dialogue between Rodrigo and Stanford. Rodrigo talks about a recent skiing trip with his wife. During the trip he had many thoughts about disaster and dying, and about his wife dying. Jonathan becomes interested and says to him, "I don't understand." Rodrigo is somewhat irritated and says, "I thought it was obvious what I was saying." Adele addresses Rodrigo and questions him about his reluctance to explain. Rodrigo is clearly cautious and negative about Adele's remark.

In the meantime for the past two sessions Arcadia's initial optimism over the group merger has changed dramatically. She has felt caught between the disapproval of one of her "allies" in her group, Julia, and is very upset with other members of Group B, especially Jonathan, whom she feels is analyzing her before knowing anything about her. In some way I feel that she is falling between the cracks during this merger. She announces that she is going to leave the group at the end of the month (this is the first session in the month). She arrived half an hour late at this session, and brought some knitting. This has been symptomatic of her behavior in the past when she is bored or anxious. I ask her, "How are you feeling, what is happening?"

She tells the group that she went home from work before coming to the group. She worried that she had left the oven on and worried about her cat. The group had talked about her being so angry the session before. As time goes on I say to her: "Your concern about the oven on may have something to do with the heat in this group the last session." She quickly responds: "No, I don't think so. You always put more into my thoughts than what they mean. I don't feel comfortable. I feel that I am starting all over again and all the progress that I had made is evaporating. Coming here tonight I felt that terrible anxiety that I used to feel like panic. I had not felt that in a long time."

I ask Ortencia, the quiet one: "What are your thoughts? Don't think too hard." She responds: "Well, I make a distinction between safety and comfort. I don't think I will gauge my staying or leaving the group on the basis of comfort. But I know I need safety to be able to talk about my anxiety, my discomforts."

Rodrigo fires another salvo and tells Arcadia (they are fond of each other) that she should have kicked Jonathan. Adele's attitude has begun to change noticeably and she talks with enthusiasm about a recent workshop she organized in a nearby city (she is a very educated woman and quite competent in her line of work). She talks about her pleasure in speaking Spanish with two other colleagues from Latin America. Alvaro talks about a coming interview for a new job and about a wonderful secret. His secret is about his own little group, his marital therapy with another analyst and me. We meet weekly the four of us and he finds him a very interesting character and is becoming more and more curious about his own reactions to him.

> Rodrigo brings us two dreams. In one he is smoking a cigarette and somebody else is also smoking with him. He knows that when the cigarette ends he is going to die. Yet he seems relieved rather than anxious.

In another dream I am in the dream filling out a form in triplicate, one is green, another yellow, and the third one white or neutral-like. His wife gets one indicating that somehow she had finished her therapy and she is okay. He then cannot find his form or the one intended for him. The whole group joins in associations to Rodrigo's dreams pointing out, among other things, that since he is not a smoker the images seem to relate to something happening in the group. After listening for some time to various comments I make the following interpretation to Rodrigo: "You have to let a penis die before you can have your actual penis. And if that can happen, even though it is a death, it is also a relief." Rodrigo thinks for a moment and then says: "I don't know exactly how, but it sounds right. I just think that what you are saying sounds right." Perhaps this is a moment of a simple truth. The group has helped me say something to a group member that appears to him quietly convincing.

Discussion

The particular group situation that I have presented can illuminate some aspects of the work with the unconscious in the psychoanalytic group. I will point out, first of all, that the changes in these groups amounted to a modification of some parameters of the analytic frame while others remained constant. Those aspects that changed were: the day of the meetings for the new group, and the membership of the new group with all of the dynamic implications: expanded possibilities for role identification and differentiation, greater stress on competitive aspects for each member and greater anxiety over issues of cohesiveness of the self, affect and behavior regulation, basic trust, belonging, identity, and capacity to maintain the therapeutic culture in the new group. Those aspects remaining constant were the same therapist, the same amount of time, the same fee, and the same therapeutic method of exploration.

Each member experienced a variety of reactions that could be summarized as follows: those from Group A (the "optimistic" group) manifested as a whole a greater degree of activity and aggression within themselves and toward Group B. Those from Group B were at the beginning more passive and even somewhat shocked and paralyzed, but gradually began to establish a place for themselves at times remarkably different from their previous one before the group merger.

I will point out some individual manifestations of the transference. From Group A: Arcadia, who originally was looking forward to the new group, becomes increasingly anxious, mistrustful, and disappointed. She asks to go back into individual therapy with me and, as announced, she leaves the group at the end of the month. She does stay for four sessions after her announcement and is able to experience some degree of challenge and respect from the group members. Julia continues flourishing, working with major life issues after divorce: changing her name, selling her home and moving to an apartment, changing careers, and continuing exploration with changes in her sexual identity. She begins to consider leaving the group. Rodrigo also begins to talk about leaving the group in a way that he has not been able to approach before this. At this point he has done what he considers a quite productive 8-year analysis with another analyst; and I have worked with him and his wife in marital psychotherapy for 5 years. He considers the marital therapy also fairly significant in positive changes, yet, after that therapy he has stayed in group therapy with me for 3 years. In his two dreams, I may be the one smoking a cigarette along with him. The form in triplicate (we were a form in triplicate: his wife green? he yellow? I white?) may represent his still unresolved struggle to leave me, whereas his wife did. As the initiator of salvos in the new group this may have to do with a movement toward the giving up of taking my place with the mother group, but not without some final attempts at smoking with me. The impending death at the end of the smoke, signals perhaps the relief of not having to be the chosen phallus and the recognition of a basic lack that can free him. Alvaro begins to talk more openly about his secret, his special relationship with another analyst and me in the marital psychotherapy. He begins to talk about having fun in therapy. At the same time, however, in one of the following weeks he forgets about his marital session, and the week after he forgets the group session. This is totally new; Alvaro never forgets about his sessions. Is this new behavior in Alvaro a manifestation of what he calls fun, meaning a capacity to be ordinary, to also forget, and not to have to be the assistant to the therapist, reminding the other members of the group attendance, being the substitute father like he had to be in his family of origin? Stanford, the youngest member from Group A, begins to get more involved with the old and new members and seems to begin to break out of his isolation. At the same time, though, he experiences great confusion and requests individual sessions in addition to the group. As for the members of Group B, Jonathan and Adele move into a new gear. Jonathan, after his initial shock, begins to have quite graphic incestuous dreams and his capacity for exploration seems to begin to rival that of Rodrigo. Adele, who appeared determined to leave the group, becomes invigorated and her depression begins to change dramatically. She declares that she likes the new group and becomes freer in the exploration of her feelings and thoughts. Ortencia, although still remaining fairly quiet, opens up more and seems to begin to come out of her shell. Belinda, however, absent for a number of sessions because of her surgery, becomes disoriented, confused and for quite a few sessions cannot move off a fairly concrete stance in the way she hears group comments. The stirred-up landscape in this new group calls my attention both to intrapsychic aspects and cultural phenomena. I find some of Lacan's methods of talking about the unconscious quite useful in understanding the communications in this new group. Let me refer, in a greatly simplified manner, to some of his concepts, before I go back to the group process.

    For Lacan the unconscious is structured like a language. This means that the unconscious is a discourse, and it is a discourse that speaks to us. It speaks to us through the linguistic forms of metaphor and metonymy, in the same ways that the dream, according to Freud, speaks to us through condensation and displacement.

This discourse that speaks to its comes from the position of an Other. This position Lacan calls transindividual. The unconscious surprises us. It manifests a basic *spaltung*, (splitting), a profound division of the subject. Furthermore, this otherness relates to the primary Other, the mother, and later on to language, to the symbolic Other, to the law of the father, through which the child enters into the oedipal, triangular relations. The child's giving up of the imaginary (narcissistic) relationship to the mother is ushered in by language. Lacan discusses at length Freud's child observation of his nephew and the words of the child *Fort . . . Da* as a key example of the function of language, and of the constitution of the subject. This step into the symbolic at the same time as it frees the child from the imaginary alienates him/her through the wall of language and leaves a permanent mark in the human being as incomplete, as divided, as always experiencing a lack of being (*manque a être*) that propels his/her desire. The recognition by the subject of his/her desire, and the naming of it, is central to Lacan's view of the function of analysis. More and more I use this as a guide to my work as a therapist. These are Lacan's words in Seminar II (published 1988).

> To bring the subject to recognize and to name his desire, this is the nature of the efficacious action of analysis. But it is not a question of recognizing something that would have already been there—a given—ready to be captured. In naming it, the subject creates, gives rise to something new, makes something new present in the world. (Book II: 228-9)

How did the unconscious desires of the members of this group come out? I will point out the following dynamics as indicators of the movement from temporary chaos to desire in the merging of the groups:

1. Personally, I had to examine several aspects of my motivation in stimulating this change, and of the dangers and potential benefits for the therapeutic work.

2. As the change got under way, seesaw movements from faith to skepticism, interest and indifference, acceptance vs. rejection, engagement vs. fleeing, love and hate, omnipotence and impotence, life and death, became apparent in the discourse of the group, in the dreams and in the acting out of some members. Some of the typical individual ego states were reenacted in the central transferences to the therapist and the group as a whole, and in the multiple transferences from member to member.

3. The positions that individual members and I each took before the announcement of the merger began to shift in some cases to exactly the opposite of the previously held convictions and attitudes.

4. Members began to find in the newcomers missing repressed qualities of themselves but also rejected, denied, and repressed bad aspects.

The partial change in the frame of these two groups as they became a new group brought up powerful repressed aspects of the unconscious. For the neurotic, the couch and warmth and comfort can be symbolic of the mother's love; for the psychotic it would be more true to say that these things are the analyst's physical expression of love. (Winnicott, 1975: 199)

Jose Bleger (1967), an Argentinean analyst, speaks of the frame in the following terms:

> A relationship which lasts for years, in which a set of norms and attitudes is kept up, is nothing less than a true definition of institution. The frame is then an institution within whose bounds certain phenomena take place, which we call behavior . . . each institution is a portion of the individual's personality, and it is of such importance that identity is always, wholly or partially, institutional in the sense that at least one part of the identity always shapes itself by belonging to a group, institution, ideology, party, etc. (1967, reprinted 1981, p. 460)

Bleger goes on to demonstrate that this organized or stable frame becomes the repository of the psychotic, symbiotic, or nondifferentiated part of the self that he also calls the non-ego or metaego. He adds that "the frame is a permanent presence, like the parents for the child. Without them, there is no development of the ego, will to keep the frame beyond necessity, or to avoid any change in the relationship with the frame or with the parents, there may be even a paralysis of development (1981, p. 464).

As I work in the psychoanalytic group I tend to think of two basic dialogues that are operating all the time. I call these dialogues, the dialogue *in* the group and thee dialogue *of* the group. The first one is along the line of consciousness; the second one is the dialogue of the unconscious. The dialogue of the unconscious cannot be apprehended directly, only by its effects, through speech, through lapses, substitutions, metaphors, jokes, etc. What were some of the pointers to the unconscious, to this Other, that can be apprehended through the discourse of the group? Looking back, I come up with a number of examples:

> "I am not going to change anyway . . ." (Adele)

> Rodrigo's salvos in the first session of the new group and Alvaro's defense of Rodrigo to the group.

> "I don't know what to say, I don't have words. . . . I am so struck by my reaction, why am I so paralyzed by Rodrigo's comments?" (Jonathan)

> Stanford growling at me and his phrase, "I have no thoughts."

> "Are you glad you are alive?" (therapist to Stanford)

> "I don't understand . . ." (Jonathan)

> "I thought it was obvious what I was saying." (Rodrigo)

"That's your sloppy work, I have given you my home address many times." (Rodrigo to therapist)

Arcadia's upset with Julia and Jonathan. Her announcement that she was to leave the group.

"How are you feeling? What is happening?" (therapist to Arcadia)

"Your concern about the oven on may have something to do with the heat in this group the last session." (therapist to Arcadia)

"You always put more into my thoughts than what they mean." (Arcadia to therapist)

"Don't think too hard." (therapist to Ortencia)

"Well, I make a distinction between safety and comfort." (Ortencia referring to Arcadia's comments)

"You should have kicked Jonathan." (Rodrigo to Arcadia)

Alvaro's pride in talking about his other small group with me and another analyst and his wife.

Stanford's and Rodrigo's theme of death and subsequent comments by the group on his dreams.

Adele letting the group know about recent success and her pleasure at speaking Spanish.

All these phrases and actions that speak have made me realize in writing this article how little I knew while in the group of the power my position and the position of the group for each member through this process. It is clearer, now, how much I was in the position of an Other for the group, and how powerful this transference was in the reawakening of conflicting desires in the group members. It is often only in retrospect that the dialogue *of* the group, the dialogue of the unconscious in the group, can be recognized, as opposed to the dialogue of consciousness, the imaginary dialogue, that can be apprehended as it happens.

The force of the repetition compulsion comes out in a number of the previous examples and points out the patients' attempts at maintaining endless possibilities at the expense of defining necessities. In other words, what the patient is trying to avoid through repetition is a simple truth. To point out the unconscious is to take a step that stops contingency to give way to what at times may appear as an "ordinary" realization—one that, however, may have far-reaching effects for the person. Jacques-Allain Miller, the editor of Lacan's writings and teachings, says it well:

> The patient develops what we could present as a sequence of words, let us call them signifiers, which appear to be infinite, potentially infinite. There is always in the narration of one's life, a strong character of

contingency. You experience your life by telling or articulating aspects of it. It was like this but it could have been like that. It was somebody, but I could have been somebody else. What have in the end is contingency. That is the meaning in logic of the possible. It happened like this, but it could have happened like that—when we discover, when you glimpse necessity in analysis—it's frequently, I won't say always, a gratifying moment for the patient. Be it hard necessity or horrible necessity, it feels like a victory over the unconscious. (1995, p. 237)

When the patient can really "see" that it was like it was and moving the curtains blinding the eyes what may appear is a simple truth ordinary and inevitable yet quietly freeing in its necessity. Lacan spoke of this necessity as something that is always being written in one's life. Analysis, then, becomes a reading, a reading of certain constants that are there all the time but need to be named. This naming and this reading are at the service of evolution. The process is in many respects a quiet revolution, one that today's techno-logical man may want to reject as too alien to this age's imaginary paradise.

Shoshna Felman, explaining Lacan and his attempt to return us to the radical discovery of Freud, writes the following:

> This is what constitutes the radicality of the Freudian unconscious, which is not simply *opposed* to consciousness—but speaks *from within* the speech of consciousness, which it subverts. The unconscious is thenceforth no longer as is it has traditionally been conceived—the simple outside of the conscious, but rather a division, *spaltung*, cleft with consciousness itself, the unconscious is no longer the difference between consciousness and the unconscious, but rather the inherent, irreducible difference between consciousness and itself. The unconscious therefore, is the radical castration of the mastery of consciousness, which turns out to be forever incomplete, illusory, and self deceptive. (1987, p. 57)

To arrive at some simple truths time and time again is the aim in the psychoanalytic group. The dialogues in the group and the dialogues of the group constitute a privileged intersubjective space that stops both the individual and the group from fully imagining that they are God, that they have infinite possibilities. Yet it is in the reading of the basic split that informs our lack of being that the individual members and the group as a whole can also find the profound desires that run like underground rivers and make humans God-like.

The Puerto Rican poet Julia de Burgos (1997) eloquently presents the dual dialogue going on in her own self. In the richness of her poetry she speaks of the same basic concept that Lacan presents when speaking of the human subject. From her poem, "To Julia de Burgos," we can hear the human paradox:

Ya las gentes murmuran que yo soy tu enemiga

porque dicen que en verso doy al mundo tu yo.

Mienten Julia de Burgos, mienten Julia de Borgos.

La que se alza en mis versos no es tu voz: es mi voz.

Porque tu eres un ropaje y la esencia soy yo;

Y el más profundo abismo se tiende entre los dos.

Already the people murmur that I am your enemy

Because they say that in verse I give the world your me.

They lie Julia de Burgos, they lie Julia de Burgos.

Who rises in my verses is not your voice: it is my voice.

Because you are the dressing and the essence is me;

And the most profound abyss is spread between us. (Translation by Jack Agüera)

Acknowledgment

Extract from the poem "To Julia de Burgos" quoted by kind permission of the publishers, Curbstone Press.

References

Bleger, J. (1967). Psychoanalysis of the psychoanalytic frame. *International Journal of Psychoanalysis, 48*, 5, 11–19.

Bleger, J. (1981). Psychoanalysis of the psychoanalytic frame. In R. Langs (Ed.), *Classics in psychoanalytic technique*. New York: Jason Aronson.

Burgos, J. de (1997). *Songs of the simple truth: The complete poems of Julia de Burgos* (Jack Agüera, Comp. & Trans.). Willimantic, CT: Curbstone Press.

Felman, S. (1987). *Jacques Lacan and the adventure of insight—Psychoanalysis in contemporary culture*. Cambridge, MA: Harvard University Press.

Lacan, J. (1988). *The seminar of Jacques Lacan, Book II: The ego in Freud's theory and in the technique of psychoanalysis: 1954–1955* (Jacques-Alain Miller, Ed.; Sylvana Tomaselli, Trans., with notes by John Forrester). New York: W. W. Norton.

Miller, J. A. (1995). Introductory talk at Sainte-Anne Hospital. In R. Feldstein, B. Fink, & M. Jaanus (Eds.), *Reading Seminar XI: Lacan's Four Fundamental Concepts of Psychoanalysis*. Albany, NY: State University of New York Press.

Winnicott, D. W. (1975). *Through pediatrics to psychoanalysis*. New York: Basic Books.

Introduction to Object Relations Group Psychotherapy

Ramon Ganzarain

Object relations group psychotherapy is one of the various group-centered psychoanalytic techniques. It focuses on the internal fantasied world of psychic reality, more specifically on the exchanges between the self and the internal images of others, or mental residues of their relations with the self. These mental representations of others—often called "internal objects"—can trigger behavioral responses, as if they were either persecutors ("bad" objects) or sources of security ("good" objects). Object relations technique makes specific use of the characteristic psychotic-like style of group mentation by focusing on the early anxieties reactivated by the regression each individual experiences when becoming a group member. Such anxieties derive mainly from conflicts with aggression in the fantasied exchanges between the self and its object, perceived as a threat, either of annihilation of the self (schizoparanoid anxiety) or of destruction of the loved objects (depressive anxiety).

Psychotic-like anxieties are very intense, imaginary, but normal threats, comparable to those felt by very sick psychiatric patients. Paranoid anxiety refers to the anticipated annihilation of the ego by powerful persecutors. The prevalent defense against it is splitting, which leads to the fragmentation of both the ego and the objects, weakening the former and making the latter appear as very threatening. By contrast, the depressive anxiety is the fear that one's own aggression could annihilate or has already destroyed one's good object. The ego feels threatened in identification with that object. After attacking an ambivalently loved mother, the self experiences losing her as an external and internal object, which gives rise to pain, guilt, and the feelings of loss. Although the intensity of these anxieties culminates during infancy, they are not exclusive of a passing phase, such as, for

example, the "oral" stage, but persist throughout life, as specific configurations—
which Klein called "positions"—of object relations, anxieties, and defenses.

The mental representations of others are either "total" or "part" objects—
according to whether they include a relatively complete or a partial picture of
the persons involved. The internal objects can also be multipersonal or collective
images, such as the images of the parental couple, of the family, of the group,
of the mother country, and so on. Group members fantasize the existence of the
"group entity," as an internal object, different from the actual collection of individuals in the room. This entity is a vaguely shared fantasy that replaces the "real"
group in the members' minds. The group as an internal object may take various
forms. Bion (1961) described it as the "basic assumptions" group. Since group
members use projective identification to defend themselves against psychotic
anxieties, each member disowns these basic assumptions, claiming no personal
participation in them, perceived as "not me," while the same individual simultaneously believes those assumptions are an active, relevant, and powerful part of
the group where he or she belongs; hence, each member perceives them also as
part of "me." In other words, the group as an object is neither self, nor other, but
both—like a transitional object (Winnicott, 1951). Since the basic assumptions
are the disowned parts of the individuals, they are anonymous, hence they may
function ruthlessly (since no one is personally responsible!), which is why members fear them.

The group as an object can become a metaphor with multiple meanings. Bion
(1961) conceptualized the basic assumptions as clusters of defenses and fantasies regarding the group as mother, reflecting her mainly as a part-object, in the
Kleinian sense, and offering a range of primitive defensive attempts to deal with
extreme anxieties. Jacobson (1989), Kossef (1990), and others view the group
entity as a "transitional phenomenon" between the self and the objects, like a
collective creation situated in Winnicott's (1967) "area of the illusion" (Jacobson,
1989). Some psychoanalysts (Modell, 1984; Rizzuto, 1979; Tolpin, 1972; Volkan,
1976) have described the human need, beyond childhood, "for relating to each
other, especially collectively, through shared representations of objects" (Jacobson, 1989, p. 480). The group entity is experienced as real and influences the
interactions between and among groupmates. It is not an abstract concept but has
a vivid psychic reality. As internal objects are projected onto other individuals in
the group, in an attempt to force them into assuming desired roles, they are also
projected onto the group entity.

It is arrived at by a process of (unspoken) negotiation in which members try
to make the group-entity what they want it to be and try to convince others that
that is what it is. In this process, everyone's negotiation strength is limited by
the need to belong to the group-entity, whatever it is (Jacobson, 1989, p. 483). It
ends up representing the objective, external group as the members desire it to be.
Those members' wishes include the need to protect the self and the loved objects
from the destruction predicted by or expected under the influence of the early
psychotic-like anxieties.

Object relations group psychotherapy techniques focus especially on the primitive defense mechanisms that shape the group-entity image, or "basic assumptions group." The primitive defense mechanisms of splitting, projective identification, omnipotent denial, projection, and introjection are the fundamental mental resources to protect the endangered self and the threatened objects from the fantasied imminent destruction. Those defenses promote fantasies of altering both the self and the objects, as well as their interactions through various identifications between the self and the object. Object relations group psychotherapy addresses those defenses and the underlying psychotic anxieties, offering the members opportunities to search for other ways to respond to their primitive fears. It conceives psychotherapeutic change as fueled by the need to resolve the depressive anxiety (the feelings of guilt) through fostering the self's capacity to repair the imaginary damages done to the loved object. Such growth of the self expands its capacity for concern, and its ability to believe and trust in the prevalence of the capacity to love over aggression (or "badness") thus integrating both poles of the ambivalence.

Some mental resources available to counteract the depressive anxieties are "manic" defenses and regression to the schizoparanoid "position" or style. Both are pathogenic because they prevent the further emotional development or ego growth stimulated by the working through of the depressive position. The manic strategy exalts the power of the self by denying both its "weakening" dependency and its guilt regarding the damaged object; the aggrandized power of the self is believed to control/dominate/devalue and triumph over its objects. The regression to the schizoparanoid position allows the self to use splitting of the self and/or of the objects to take refuge against anxiety in the relationship with an idealized, omnipotently good object image; this strategy enhances the power of the protecting object to alleviate the persecutory anxiety awakened by the "bad" ones.

The overcoming of the manic defenses and of the regression to a schizoparanoid position is a prerequisite to effective psychotherapeutic work. Otherwise, manic denial prevents the realization that something is wrong and needs to be amended. If a member feels that everything is wonderful, there is no motivation for change! Likewise, if patients feel that someone else should be blamed (the paranoid stance) for their sufferings, they will not make any therapeutic effort and would rather turn away (schizoid attitude) from the relationship with the group.

Other group-centered psychoanalytic techniques do not focus on the primitive defense mechanisms' struggles against psychotic-like anxieties. Neither Ezriel's (1951) search for the "common group tension," Whitaker and Lieberman's (1964) group "focal conflict" approach, Horwitz's (1977) "group-centered technique," nor Agazarian and Peters's (1981) "systems" conceptualization deal with these early anxieties and defenses, although all focus on group-as-a whole phenomena. Although Horwitz (1983) conceives of projective identification as an important defense mechanism, he does not examine it in the context of the incipient ego's struggles against psychotic-like anxieties. By contrast, what is unique to object relations group psychotherapy is that the patients often experience this theory's concepts as the "natural language" to verbalize and to communicate their feelings, anxieties, and fantasies regarding their internalized relationships, including those with the group entity. Thus, the operating concepts of this theory may open up to therapeutic explorations, the whole range of psychopathological expressions of the psychotic-like anxieties, including those of persons not clinically insane.

Although object relations group psychotherapy focuses mostly on the vicissitudes of the group entity, it does not exclude intrapsychic or interpersonal components of the group life. Each member's intrapsychic struggles are addressed as a common conflict shared in various degrees by all members. Some researchers of the effectiveness of group-centered treatments have described how some individuals feel abandoned because the attention of the therapist is focused on group issues. These complaints of patients, who felt frustrated, have been misused to discredit the group-centered modalities of group psychotherapy because they induce the narcissistic injury of some members. However, the angry deprivation can instead be used to explore the ambivalent relationship with the group entity as a maternal surrogate. In addition, the intrapsychic issues (Parloff, 1968) of each member are in many regards like those of the groupmates. Similarities among members give comfort and provide mirrors to look at one's self. Exploration of individual peculiarities can also be privately done within each person's mind, while choosing what, when, and whether to talk about them during the group meetings.

Clinical Illustrations

I shall describe here some clinical observations of outpatient groups in their working phase*; the members were not psychotic, although some were borderline and narcissistic personalities. When indicated, I shall sparingly insert brackets documenting my theoretical constructs. But if the reader wishes to follow the main flow of ideas better, those brackets may first be ignored and read later on, if necessary. I shall begin this section by reporting on a group working on initial shared resistances as defenses against the increment of psychotic anxieties during the first ten sessions.

Hypomanic Defenses: Pairing and Acting Out
This clinical illustration is a summary of the ninth session of an outpatient group formed by four women and four men all married, white, and middle class (Ganzarain, 1991); among them, four were "difficult to treat"; they met twice a week for 75 minutes at the Menninger Foundation Audiovisual Studio.

Rose was absent for the second time. During the first half of meeting 9, Judith, the youngest and most attractive female, spoke about her sexual difficulties, vaginismus, and frigidity, which had made her first 2 years of marriage

---

* In object relations group psychotherapy, the analysis of psychotic-like anxieties (derived from conflicts with aggression) is focused from the start on the group expressions of hostility; in that regard, the "work" phase begins earlier than in other psychoanalytic modes.

nearly impossible to endure. The group discussed her situation, asked pertinent questions, and suggested additional treatment measures. I will now focus in detail on the second half of this meeting, after Roland shared that he was having an extramarital affair because his sexual needs were not satisfied with his wife. He proceeded to describe a Don Juan-like sexual life, adding his feelings of guilt for having to lie to his wife, but also his unwillingness to change his sexual behavior. Male members responded with criticism. Judith reacted with worried curiosity inquiring "If you are not pleased with your wife, then why do you stay married?" For her, Roland's infidelity was exactly what she feared most from her husband due to her own sexual dysfunctions.

Secretly, however, Roland seized this moment to talk about his sexual life in part as a response to Judith's sharing her marital difficulties. It was as if he were saying to her, "Do you need a sexual 'expert'? I can help you." Thus presenting himself personally to her as an alleged sexual expert, he attempted to pair with Judith.

Cathy revealed that she was also having an affair behind her spouse's back. Cathy elaborated on feeling guilty and trying to push men away from her by becoming overweight, while on the other hand starving for the emotional gratification of sexual intimacy. She stated, "I do not do it for the sex, but for the love," to counteract [use of sex to "deny"] depression and loneliness. She did not want to dump on her husband all the many "rotten things" that she felt she contained. There were further group criticisms for those cheating on their spouses. However, the group members gradually moved to understand them: What was the psychological explanation of their extramarital affairs? By now Roland and Cathy had become like another "pair," united by the group's current attention to their sexual lives. Maybe they wanted to get back at their spouses because they were angry at them? Most certainly they were afraid of losing the spouses [depressive anxiety]. Daniel, whose wife had threatened divorce, was sure that was their case. Another member concurred. Judith thought they did it because of sexual frustration. Daniel insisted, "I am afraid my wife will be gone any day!" Suddenly this brought an experience to Cathy's mind; she burst into tears and said, "That's it. I'm afraid of losing him as I lost my father! That's it!" She then proceeded to tell the group about her father's suicide. He killed himself when he was 42. He had been an alcoholic and had gone to AA meetings. His two sober months were interrupted by a relapse into drinking. He killed himself after this relapse. Group members gradually shared their feelings that loved persons could also abruptly leave them. They asked for details about the suicide of Cathy's father. Roland said, "There is a curious parallelism: My father was a 'control-aholic' who couldn't relax. He saw me doing 'meditation exercises,' learning to relax, and he wanted to learn them. I taught him, but he could not stand what he discovered within himself. He lost his mind and killed himself shortly after." Some members exclaimed, "Oh my God!" The group's oldest man then started reflecting about his own vulnerability; he reported that he felt tremendously vulnerable particularly with his wife. He wanted to understand how one could become so vulnerable. He pointedly addressed this question to the therapist.

This question marked a significant change in the style of interacting with the therapist during this session. In the second half of this meeting I was literally excluded, silenced by the frantic rhythm of exchanges among members. When the oldest man asked about his vulnerability, I was in a dilemma. There were only 3 more minutes left to conclude the session, but important material had emerged; the group was now asking me to comment. I decided to intervene saying that becoming involved in the group was making them vulnerable to the fear of losing or missing each other and perhaps that was why they had not inquired about Rose's absence. I also reminded the group that upon convening the previous meeting, Roland had shared the information that psychiatrists are the professionals with the highest rate of suicide. Some members spontaneously interrupted, saying, "The group will be gone too [the group entity]! Or you may be gone!" Judith was then crying. The therapist briefly added, "There is a fear of the responsibility of harming someone [depressive anxiety], maybe Rose, the missing member? Or perhaps driving me to become suicidal." A brief silence followed. Roland said (to the therapist), "When you were talking, I had the impulse to stand up and start giving a hug to everyone in the room." Cathy responded immediately with loud laughter [hypomanic reaction] and said, "Oh yeah!" Judith was still crying.

The therapist's remarks first brought a brief moment of reflection, with Judith crying and others acknowledging their fears that the group or the therapist might be gone forever. But shortly after, the group's hypomanic defenses were reinforced, and there was again a brief plan to "become physically intimate" by hugging. It was significant that Roland proposed the idea and that Cathy immediately endorsed it. The two "acting outers" had briefly "acted in" their defensive styles in dealing with depression! The group had previously indulged in pseudointimacy through "talking about sex," as if the topic would bring them closer, without having to pay attention to their fears of hurting each other. Significantly the subject of the meeting's second half was "casual sex" used to fill in the void of depression and to forget anxiety. Anxiety was, however, significantly present with unconscious worries about the group's survival, as if members were feeling, "If one patient misses a session will this mean that she will later on drop out and then others may do the same? Have we hurt Rose, the missing member?" Or the other way around: "If I get more involved here, would I be hurt? I risk losing persons that I may need here." The group's anxiety about its survival was defended against by the pairing basic assumption, expressed as a hope that members could help each other to overcome the fears of love being hurtful. Similar expectations about the omnipotent "cure-it-all" magic quality of love had also inspired Roland's and Cathy's acting out.

During most of the session, I was perceived as a threat. The treatment could make them face the truth about themselves, as the AA meetings might have contributed to Cathy's father's suicide, or as the truth discovered during meditation exercises had pushed Roland's father into madness and suicide! The therapist had become in their minds like the sphinx: a silent witness whose knowledge had killing powers. I was, off and on, perceived then unconsciously as the persecutor [paranoid anxiety] that group members had to eliminate because I knew too much. In other moments, they projected into me their own vulnerability, their potential for suicidal depression, and were fighting with a sense of guilt for wishing to harm me lethally.

The group's request for my intervention probably was an attempt to restore or repair, by implication, and thus relieve the patients' fears of me, by listening to my comments and realizing with relief that I was intact, "all right." In addition, my references to their most intense anxieties soothed them, albeit briefly, making them feel understood.

The destructive potential of sadomasochistic exchanges (between Judith and her husband, between Cathy's and Roland's families and their fathers, as well as between the group and Rose) needed to be "manically" denied, proclaiming instead the alleged omnipotence of love by engaging in pseudocaring interactions, thus attempting to create an atmosphere of hope within the group. The two main topics of the ninth meeting had been "love hurts" (illustrated by Judith's vaginismus) and "intimacy makes you vulnerable" (i.e., Daniel's fear of losing his wife); both topics expressed fears about closeness among persons in the group, possibly causing its disintegration. Instead of talking about these anxieties, the members attempted to develop an atmosphere of pseudointimacy by talking about sex and tentatively exploring possible heterosexual couples within the group, as if trying to again use pseudoerotic "actions" to allay the primitive psychotic-like anxieties of being attacked/eliminated [paranoid fears] or of driving someone to commit suicide [depressive]. The therapist's linking the outside issues such as hurtful sex, philandering, fathers' suicides, and so on, to the [here-and-now] group events—such as hurting members' vulnerability, information about psychiatrists' high rate of suicide, fear of losses, and so on—served as a role model regarding how to examine and how to talk about deep anxieties instead of avoiding them, as well as how to understand some attempted ineffectual solution of these primitive fears. Some members (Judith, Daniel) utilized the therapeutic comments to acknowledge their fears and felt understood by the therapist; Roland and Cathy transiently reinforced instead their usual defenses, almost resorting again to action; by wishing to "act in" hugging everyone, they again displayed their action-oriented response to their basic anxieties.

The timing of my intervention deserves some comments. I took the opportunity offered to me, feeling that the group needed—above all—to hear from me that I was all right, neither hurt, vengeful, nor suicidal. Then it was very important for them to verify that I was okay! The realization that I was still all right was more important than the content of whatever I had to say, because during the session they had left me out and turned away from me. I felt "left out" as a counter-transferential response to their transference to me, casting me in the role of the feared, despised, and yet needed spouse. Verifying my tolerance for their hurting me became a significant need for the members' reassurance against their fears of me as vengeful [paranoid anxiety]. I elected to focus my comments at the level of the group-centered issues: by examining the consecutive absences of the member probably hurt by the group's hostility as forecasting the possible disintegration of the group, connecting it with how love hurts, making a person vulnerable, even crazy or suicidal. The members' fears of being hurt back [persecutory fears] and/or deserted by the vengeful therapist/spouse/father/group entity were another source of the common group tension requiring my attention. Simultaneously some intrapsychic and interpersonal (Parloff, 1968) issues were also implicitly touched upon, like Cathy's and Roland's complex intense feelings regarding their fathers' suicide or the older member warning the others about his vulnerability.

Working Through a Melancholic-Like Anxiety
Let me now turn to clinical material from another more advanced group. Nine students about to graduate from professional schools of the University of Chile had been functioning as a psychotherapeutic group, meeting once a week for 90 minutes in my private office. Eight (three women and five men, four married and four single) were resuming their regular meetings after a summer break; previously they had met for 42 sessions. One member, Joe, had already graduated from the group as well as from the university, and had taken a job and entered private practice in another city. The group was then facing three problems: (1) the loss of Joe, a very active and popular member; (2) the possibility of bringing in a new member; and (3) an annual raise in their fees on account of severe inflation. I will focus on the participation of Peter, another member in the group.

Peter missed Joe and described how Joe had been very important for him. He said, "I have difficulties in expressing my hostility and I identified myself with Joe. He spoke for me." He added that through identifying himself with Joe he was also getting the therapist's attention and affection. Peter was the spokesman for the group's emotional reaction to the loss of one of its most popular members. Sensing a mood of depression, I helped them to link the loss of their most popular member with the fear of the end of the group's existence. Although the group members had ambivalent relationships with Joe, they denied their hostility toward him and idealized him. Another member talked about a situation in which he felt guilty because he had taken over somebody's job. Although other members reassured him, the therapist interpreted that they felt guilty about the possibility or wish of taking over Joe's function within the group because it was like making him disappear and that they were now experiencing guilt [depressive anxiety] over their greed to "incorporate" or take over somebody's role. Under those circumstances, they began perceiving the therapist as greedy for money, and now they were angry at him because of his policy of yearly raising the fees following the rate of inflation. The group expressed several metaphors in oral sadistic terms such as being devoured, exploited, emptied by this greedy therapist, who was about to deprive them of many "goodies" by raising their fees. At this point I interpreted the projective meaning of their perception of hint; that is, they were avoiding acknowledging that they themselves were greedy in wanting to take over Joe's and the therapist's roles in the group.

In the following session two members identified themselves with Joe [the lost object] in a different way by considering the possibility of dropping out of the group. In response, other members acknowledged that they had felt abandoned by the doctor during his recent summer vacation. Peter pointed out that the group was important for him, but he had realized that both he and the others tended to deny the group's importance [group entity] and to derogate it by resorting to humor. Furthermore, they devalued the group as a way of defending themselves against feeling sad or deprived, because they had missed each other or the therapist while on vacation. When they started to acknowledge that they missed each other, there was a very active interchange of cigarettes and matches among the members. All of them started simultaneously to smoke. While they were grabbing cigarettes from each other, one of them commented sarcastically, "You see we don't need each other; we don't need love from the other members." Peter then took a leading role within the group and acted as a therapist by focusing the group's attention on Paul's behavior, mainly on his inhibition. Paul tried to relate his inhibition to his family's low socioeconomic background: he elaborated that when he started attending the university he only had one suit, one overcoat, one pair of shoes, and so forth. Paul reminded the group that he was born after his oldest brother had died, that he was a replacement child named after the deceased sibling. There was a family myth about how handsome and clever the oldest brother was. I commented that Paul must have felt as if he were a thief who had stolen his brother's identity, occupying a place in which he did not belong. Peter commented on Paul's excessive worrying about the amount of attention he was getting from the group and the amount of time that was being devoted to him. Other members reminded Paul that when he had had an opportunity for a promotion at work (because of the departure of his chief, whose job he took), Paul had felt very uncomfortable. He elaborated on his constant feeling of having displaced someone.

I would like to emphasize how Peter was leading the group in accomplishing its therapeutic task with Paul: helping him to realize the inappropriateness of his underestimating himself and relating his inhibition to his guilt about his greediness. Guilt was making Paul feel responsible for stealing the central role in the group. In the same way, he felt he had stolen his previous chief's job and his eldest brother's identity. While helping Paul to master his inhibition, Peter himself was overcoming the same conflict through his own activity in the group. Peter was now confident enough to take on the therapist's functions within the group, as well as to occupy Joe's previous role.

The next session, Paul came remarkably better dressed; in addition, he told the group that after he had thought over the previous session, he realized how he devalued himself by his constant comparison with the idealized image of his dead brother. He also reported that he had had a series of nightmares. In all of them the central character was a 10-year-old child, who was in reality his nephew, the current "child of the family." While taking care of that child, the boy's life was suddenly in danger from an earthquake. Paul was unable to run, to inform someone about the danger the child was in, or to rescue him. Ever since that dream, he had been scared and anxious (about harming a loved object). Coming back to the present Paul suddenly wondered why he had again been doing most of the talking in the group. He apologized saying that he did not want to lose the group's attention. He related his family's current pampering of his nephew to the way he assumed they might have treated his oldest brother. Paul emphasized that his fear, in the nightmare, was not that something wrong might happen to him; his main concern was how to protect the child. Several members praised Peter for his job as a therapist. Peter responded immediately that he shared this problem with Paul, also tending to express his hostility in an indirect way only.

In this clinical material (Ganzarain, 1983, p. 285) there were several instances of working through a melancholic-like anxiety. Guilt centered on losing a loved object through fantasies of greedily wishing to "devour" and to "incorporate" that object's role. These guilt feelings were mainly elaborated around Joe's departure from the group and the wish expressed by several other members (ambivalence about the loved object) to take over Joe's role and function within the group. Peter and Paul reacted in that way to Joe's departure. Patients expressed guilt, too, about taking over the therapist's role. Several members verbalized their concerns about having taken over somebody's role, both in their working situations or in their families. The working through of this guilt around fantasies of having "devoured" the role and functions of a loved object led the group members to work through some of the depressive anxieties connected with previously experienced mourning processes. The self of several members was reliving the ambivalence that each one experienced before with meaningful past objects, repeating a style of relationship where guilt prevailed, making them feel responsible for the fantasied damages caused to loved objects.

The melancholic-like guilt around greediness—an expression of oral sadism—was experienced by Paul around getting the group's attention when he described as "eating up all the group's time," while talking about his relationship with his dead brother. Other members were able to examine their guilt at asking for love and attention, both in the group and in their out-of-the-group lives.

There were several primitive, psychotic-like defense mechanisms mobilized against these depressive or melancholic-like anxieties. Greed and hostility were split and projected as a defense against guilt. Manic defenses were also operating: Dependence and guilt were denied, therapy was humorously devalued, and some considered dropping out, implying that they did not need or value the group. Through dealing with these defenses the patients were able to experience guilt and integrate their previously split and projected parts. They moved from intrapsychic fragmentation to personal integration. This integration also brought out increased group cohesiveness: they worked harder to achieve their therapeutic tasks. The group cohesiveness promotes good psychotherapeutic work in an atmosphere of warm natural support, cementing the group's working alliance and permitting members to interact as each other's therapists. While this common task is performed, the hostility inside the group evaporates, and concern then occupies center stage. As Unamuno (1951), the Spanish existentialist philosopher, wrote: "To love is to feel compassion . . . and if pleasure makes bodies one, sorrow brings souls together" (p. 851).

The patients tolerated their guilt over their oral sadistic impulses, accepting their responsibility for their hostile fantasies without disowning them through projection. Objects became, therefore, separate, differentiated individuals, and not mere containers of split parts.

The patients' view of reality was also modified. They developed a sense of psychic reality by acknowledging both dependence and ambivalence toward their objects. They modified their belief in the omnipotence of destructive and loving impulses. They discovered and practiced actual ways of affecting external reality through the hard work of reparation, accompanied by effective therapeutic interchanges.

By presenting first Peter's claims for help and later Paul's, the members were dealing with their depressive anxieties by resorting to a dependency basic assumption, putting it at the service of the work group, performing their primary therapeutic task.

The dependency basic assumptions form a cluster of defenses against guilt induced by greed. Greed is an expression of oral sadism. It is manifested in groups by behaviors that mean, "We want more." Groups try to get by force what they want from the therapist through manipulative, exploitative maneuvers. However, this group displayed appropriate dependency, which led to the members realistically assimilating the help I offered and integrating it to foster their further emotional growth. I again focused my attention in these sessions mainly on group-centered issues such as (1) the loss of Joe and the ensuing member's mourning; (2) the "manic" denial of missing the group and the therapist, devaluing their emotional importance and humorously triumphing over needing both, so that they almost did not experience during the summer break any longing to return, and some of them were even considering dropping out; (3) the related fear of the possible loss of the whole group through premature termination; and (4) the examination of the inhibition to take over the mourned lost object's role in the group [reenactment in the here and now of the there and then], in the family, or at work, which allowed the members to practice their ability to do effective reparation of the damaged object—Peter started examining Paul's inhibition to take over Joe's role, thus Paul understood and modified his guilt about his greediness for his wish to steal Joe's central role, Peter was simultaneously overcoming the same conflict by practicing his capacity to do reparation through his own "therapist-like activity" regarding Paul. Depressive anxieties of damaging a loved object, manic defenses against those fears, and the resolution of the implicit conflicts by practicing reparation were all experienced starting in these three sessions and later on worked through by this group. Through examining their primitive defenses of denial, splitting, and projection these patients became able to experience guilt instead of denying it and to integrate previously split and projected parts of themselves. They progressed to further personal integration and experienced a new sense of emotional enrichment, informed by a more complete reappraisal of their various inner resources, together with feeling a grateful responsibility and concern for their objects of love.

Discussion and Future Development

I shall now discuss the likely future of object relations group psychotherapy regarding (1) some desirable theoretical refinements and (2) the problems in the professional practice of this modality.

Theoretical Refinements

Object relations theory is both developmental and clinical, yet its terminology seems as complicated as if it were "metapsychological." This theory is focused on early emotional development and based on clinical psychoanalytic observations of children and adults. It has systematically described the primitive mental defense mechanisms and how they can prevent or alter the normal course of emotional development. However, the terminology designating its basic concepts often abuses analogy, such as when describing the developmental stages in psychopathological terms, like "schizoparanoid" or "depressive." These overdone comparisons create a confusing paradox for the student of these theories, who may find absurd that emotional growth be described as reaching the "depressive" position. A student not familiar with the Kleinian meaning of this term may wonder why, to become emotionally healthy, a patient must first experience an emotional illness like "depression." Therefore, in order to understand the object relations theory's contributions to psychotherapy, it is necessary to distinguish the actual Kleinian descriptions of the psychodynamics of psychoses from the analogies between the normal infant's developmental struggles and the functional psychoses.

Some say we now are in the age of narcissism, while others report seeing more "difficult-to-treat" patients than before. Group psychoanalytic therapy with an object relations orientation seems tailor-made to understand and treat these difficult patients, since the essential problem in dealing with narcissistic and borderline patients is their intense hostile transference. Many of those who treated these patients (Kernberg, 1968, 1974; Kohut, 1968, 1971; Rosenfeld, 1979) tried to deflect the so-called negative transference by focusing these patients' hostility occurring somewhere else, outside the group, either in a different moment or in another relationship, instead of bringing it immediately to the here and now of the therapeutic relationship. Rosenfeld (1979) advised not to "shove back" the patient's projected "bad" contents by not interpreting projection in the transference when anger had reached the "white heat" level of paranoid distortions. He waited instead for coming therapeutic sessions, when the patient's observing ego had regained its reality assessment. Rosenfeld (1979) observed that if projection was interpreted while the patient was extremely paranoid, it would likely lead to a therapeutic impasse. In group psychoanalytic therapy the therapist and the group can become the containers (Bion, 1967) of the patient's anger by giving a vivid example of how to cope with such hostility without retaliation; they can provide surrogate "good mothering" through a meaningful experience of being understood and cared for even when angry. The patient may describe current perceptions of the persons in the group, without having his or her projections immediately interpreted. The therapist can instead encourage the fellow patients to examine what they may have done wrong to the member now suffering from paranoid distortions. Such ensuing discussions may help the disturbed patient to acknowledge how his or her perceptions and judgments were transiently altered by fear or anger. Winnicott's contributions to psychoanalysis often seem to rectify, expand, and supplement Klein's (1952) original concepts, making them even more meaningful when treating difficult patients. Winnicott's theoretical formulations have also obvious connections with Kohut's self-psychology (1968, 1971), although they are not always acknowledged. The focus on the self as developing in the context of real and fantasized interrelationships, from infancy on, is at the core of object relations group psychotherapy. Its future may be further enriched by combining these different but closely related viewpoints.

There is also a trend toward theoretical expansion by acknowledging the phenomenology of "chaos" as applicable to the human mind. Our mental life is undergoing constant chaotic interactions among the part components of our mental system, so that some minor "bangs" (vaguely comparable to the big one experienced by the universe) can happen; our intuition can grasp such new organizing mental synthesis, provided we learn how to tolerate the ambiguity of unstructured mental chaos. Contemporary psychoanalytic theory is beginning to be influenced by the so-called "chaos theory" (Gleick, 1987). The complete unpredictability of chaos reigns sometimes instead of the predictability of order! So it is possible that our deepening comprehension of chaos may enrich our understanding of the human mind in its social contexts.

Problems in the Professional Practice
The group psychotherapy field has become more complex and confusing, growing in many directions. Scheidlinger (1982) describes how it has become very difficult to agree on a definition of it. Such confusion contributes to obscuring the professional status of group psychotherapists. Theoretical and technical divisions make them easy prey for the exploitative policies of some U.S. health organizations. Efforts to define the field and have the expertise of group psychotherapists fully acknowledged by educational, professional, and licensing organizations and financial institutions are desirable goals for the future of professionals practicing group psychotherapy.

Scheidlinger (1982) proposes a dear distinction among "people-helping" groups, describing four major categories: (1) group psychotherapy, (2) therapeutic groups for clients in mental health settings, (3) training and human development groups, and (4) self-help and mutual help groups. He defines group psychotherapy as a specific field of clinical practice, within the realm of the psychotherapists, a psychosocial process, wherein an expert psychotherapist with special additional group process training, utilizes the emotional interaction in small, carefully planned groups to "repair" mental ill health, that is, to effect amelioration of personality dysfunctions in individuals specifically selected for this purpose (p. 7).

   Scheidlinger describes as "therapeutic groups" all other approaches utilized by human services personnel (not necessarily trained professionals) in outpatient or inpatient facilities; often they are only auxiliary missions to another primary treatment of psychiatric patients. Distinguishing them from other group practitioners is highly desirable. The development of more training opportunities for new generations of such experts should follow. Group psychotherapy can ideally be acknowledged as a subspecialty within clinical or medical psychology. The possibility of combining group psychotherapy as the main psychological treatment with additional supplementary psychopharmacological medications may also be accepted. Ideally, however, such medications should be prescribed by a psychiatrist (other than the group psychotherapist), acting as a medication consultant, to avoid a confusion of roles and purposes, while at the same time offering the benefits of such combined approach to those patients who need it (Ganzarain, 1989).

   Some specific limitations arise in the practice of object relations group psychotherapy. Because the working through of character pathology is an essential feature, the duration of this treatment modality is bound to be long-term. Because of some "traditional" strong opposition to "Kleinian" ideas, often misrepresented as "wild analysis," there are relatively few places in the United States (Washington, D.C., certain parts of New York, Topeka, San Francisco, Los Angeles, and a few others) where this and group psychotherapy are taught and practiced. Therefore, professionals interested in learning this modality have relatively limited possibilities.

References

Agazarian, Y., & Peters, R. (1981). *The visible and the invisible group.* London: Tavistock/Routledge.

Bion, W. (1961). *Experiences in groups.* London: Tavistock.

Enid, H. (1950). A psychoanalytic approach to group treatment. *British Journal of Medical Psychology, 23,* 59–74.

Ezriel, H. (1951). The scientific testing of psycho-analytic findings and theory. *British Journal of Medical Psychology, 24*(1), 30–34.

Ganzarain, R. (1983). Working through in analytic group psychotherapy. *International Journal of Group Psychotherapy, 33,* 281–296.

Ganzarain, R. (1989). Object relations group psychotherapy. *The group as an object, as a tool, and as a training base.* Madison, CT: International Universities Press.

Ganzarain, R. (1991). The "bad" mother-group. In S. Tuttman (Ed.), *Psychoanalytic group theory and technique* (pp. 157–173). Madison, CT: International Universities Press.

Gleick, J. (1987). *Chaos: Making a new science.* New York Viking Press.

Horwitz, L. (1977). A group-centered approach to group psychotherapy. *International Journal of Group Psychotherapy, 27,* 423–440.

Horwitz, L. (1983). Projective identification in dyads and groups. *International Journal of Group Psychotherapy, 33,* 259–279.

Jacobson, L. (1989). The group as an object in the cultural field. *International Journal of Group Psychotherapy, 39,* 475–497.

Kernberg, O. (1968). The treatment of patients with borderline personality organization. *International Journal of Psychoanalysis, 49*, 600–619.

Kernberg, O. (1974). Further contributions to the treatment of narcissistic personalities. *International Journal of Psychoanalysis, 55*, 215–240.

Klein, M. (1952). Notes on some schizoid mechanisms. In J. Riviere (Ed.), *Developments in psychoanalysis* (pp. 292–320). London: Hogarth Press.

Kohut, H. (1968). The psychoanalytic treatment of narcissistic personality disorder. *Psychoanalytic Study of the Child, 23*, 86–113.

Kohut, H. (1971). *Analysis of the self.* New York: International Universities Press.

Kossef, J. W. (1990). Anchoring the self through the group: Congruences, play, and the potential for change. In B. Roth, W. Stone, & H. Kibel (Eds.), *The difficult patient in group* (pp. 87–108). Madison, CT: International Universities Press.

Modell, A. (1984). *Psychoanalysis in a new context.* New York: International Universities Press.

Parloff, M. (1968). Analytic group psychotherapy. In J. Marmor (Ed.), *Modern psychoanalysis* (pp. 492–531). New York: Basic Books.

Rizzuto, A. M. (1979). *The birth of the living god.* Chicago: University of Chicago Press.

Rosenfeld, H. (1979). Transference psychoses in the borderline patient. In J. Le Boit & A. Capponi (Eds.), *Advances in psychotherapy of the borderline patient* (pp. 485–510). New York: Jason Aronson.

Scheidlinger, S. (1982). *Focus on group psychotherapy.* New York: International Universities Press.

Tolpin, M. (1972). In the beginning of a cohesive self. *Psychoanalytic Study of the Child, 26*, 316–355.

Unamuno, M. (1951). *On the tragic sentiment of life (Del sentimiento tragico de la vida).* In Essays. Madrid: Aguilar.

Volkan, V. (1976). *Primitive internalized object relations.* New York: International Universities Press.

Whitaker, D., & Lieberman, M. (1964). *Psychotherapy through the group process.* New York: Atherton.

Winnicott, D. W. (1951). Transitional objects and transitional phenomena. In *Playing and reality* (pp. 1–50). Harmondsworth, England: Penguin, 1974.

Winnicott, D. W. (1967). The location of cultural experiences. In *Playing and reality* (pp. 112–121). Harmondsworth, England: Penguin, 1974.

Winnicott, D. W. (1971). The use of an object and relating through identifications. In *Playing and reality* (pp. 101–111). Harmondsworth, England: Penguin, 1974.

Interpersonal Approaches

The interpersonalist point of view has a certain primacy at the Washington School of Psychiatry. The School had been founded in 1936 by Harry Stack Sullivan, whose lasting contribution to today's dynamic therapy is contained in his theories of interpersonal psychology. This chapter will perforce include many offerings, all within this theoretical umbrella.

Isaiah Zimmerman's overview of this aspect of interpersonalism could well function as a basic practical explanation. It should be of interest to know that, after a long career in the clinical practice of group psychotherapy using this model, Dr. Zimmerman now applies it to large group consultations. He works with government, business, and other agencies to ensure that the interpersonal issues he delineates here are harnessed in the service of the agency's mission.

Throughout her teaching at the Washington School, Maryetta Andrews-Sachs, LCSW, has been a continual exponent of the need for any therapist, of whatever theoretical ilk, to attend thoughtfully to her/his own anxiety. Her most comprehensive statement of this position is found in the introduction she gave to the first conference on interpersonalist approaches, "Anxiety, Courage and Healing."

The final selection offered is a comprehensive theoretical discussion of this approach by Molyn Leszcz, MD. Dr. Leszcz was a frequent guest presenter at the Institute, providing perspectives on both interpersonal and existential themes. His paper "The Interpersonal Model of Group Psychotherapy" was initially presented at the Institute in somewhat different form.

George Saiger

Interpersonal Group Psychotherapy

Isaiah M. Zimmerman

Basic Concepts of the Interpersonal Approach

The history of ideas behind interpersonal group psychotherapy includes the views of Sandor Ferenczi, who passionately challenged the aloofness of the analyst's role current at his time; Franz Alexander, who introduced the term "corrective emotional experience"; and Carl Rogers, who first paid attention to accurate attunement to the patient's message and applied it in his counseling groups—and then, primarily, Harry Stack Sullivan. Sullivan first defined psychotherapy as a science of interpersonal living. He described psychiatry as being concerned with events or processes in which the [therapist] participates while being observant. He spoke of events in interpersonal fields that include the psychiatrist, not events that he looks at from atop ivory towers. He wrote that both parties interview each other, that observing one person's feelings about the other's attitudes were central to the process of psychotherapy. He held that empathy was an interpersonal process. Sullivan's attention to the immediacy of the dyadic interaction actually foreshadowed what we today call the here-and-now approach. He indicated that no two people can talk to each other without influencing each other. He said that there is always an interaction between the interviewer and the interviewee and that from it, both must invariably learn. Thus, interpersonal learning became a modality of treatment. Sullivan emphasized the universality of people's problems in living, and that transference (which he called "parataxic distortion") occurs daily to everyone. He moved therapy from a supposedly objective stance by a psychiatrist to an interpersonal process aimed at reducing perceptual distortions. Though he himself never engaged in group treatment, his ideas were eventually picked up and applied by Irvin Yalom, who is known to all of you for his

interactional approach to group. Yalom cites Sullivan extensively and sympatheti-
cally, with the comment that "Sullivan's professional fate has been similar to that
of many another innovator. The conservative community responded to his ideas
at first by ignoring them, then by attacking them, and finally by so assimilating
them that their innovative nature was forgotten" (Yalom, 1995). Nonetheless, the
integrative, interpersonal treatment approach did spread throughout much of the
mental health field. It carried with it certain key concepts: The importance of
interpersonal relationships; the structure of a corrective emotional experience;
the group as a social microcosm; the wide (but never exclusive) use of a "here and
now," jargon-free dialogue, and a therapist who acts both as a participant and an
observer (Yalom, 1995; Leszcz, 1992).

The interpersonal field holds that just as there is no baby as such, but always
a mother-child dyad (Winnicott, 1965), so is there no singular person who is not
linked up with a wide matrix of groups at all times. Pines (1996) has written that
"the individual identity of each one of us is constituted by intrapsychic, interpersonal and transpersonal processes; the boundaries of the individual extend
far beyond those of the corporeal Self." Psychological damage, when inflicted,
quickly spreads through the human network of relations. Like the Internet, we are
all ultimately attached. This audience does not need to be reminded of the centrality of disturbed interpersonal relations and that traumatization is only undone
by specific person-to-person and group reparative work, within a secure relationship and with sufficient time to work through all the stages. Medicine can help,
but it is not enough. There really is no substitute for what we do by structured and
dedicated relationship work.

Let us now look at an instance of a "Corrective Emotional Experience," in
my own group work. I normally do some initial didactic orientation with each
prospective member of a group, in addition to discussing a group contract. The
new group member gradually forms alliances and joins one or more subgroups.
I also gradually reinforce certain norms, such as having respect for each other;
that we try to understand our emotional effect upon each other and the whole
group; and that nonjudgmental curiosity about each other's thoughts, feelings, and
behavior is definitely on the agenda. At the same time, I convey the message that a
person's pace of involvement will be respected. And finally that abusive, demeaning, or threatening words or behavior are not acceptable, whereas strong feelings
are. As the new member spends more time in the group, she learns about a few
other facilitative techniques and sees them demonstrated. One is called "Listening With a Non-Rebutting Mind." Here patients learn to slow down and do their
best not to immediately engage in oppositional or argumentative thought when
they are asked to listen with a non-rebutting mind. Another skill is to "replicate"
what someone has said to you, in an effort to increase understanding. These tools
are used periodically, sometimes with some humor; and they begin to be picked
up by the new member. Despite the apparent intrusiveness and didactic flavor of
these communication aids, the group absorbs them and they are employed only on
occasion. Otherwise, they would lose their usefulness, I believe.

Here is an illustration of a corrective emotional experience in an ongoing group:

Dana, a married lawyer, after about three months in the group, began to avoid looking at me or speaking to me. He was a very experienced analytic patient who had been referred by his psychiatrist to "round out his therapy and reduce his tenseness around people." After ascertaining for a few sessions that indeed he was avoiding any contact with me, I did what I usually do. I used the subgroup he was part of at the time. I turned to them (a man and a woman, June and Tom) and asked if they could verify what I believed was going on. They said yes, and that they had recently talked about it with Dana in the parking lot. June and Tom urged Dana to talk to me. Dana kept looking at the window throughout this encounter, with a tense expression. After a moderately long silence, Dana said "I came to you because my psychiatrist strongly recommended you. And I see you're pretty good and I'll probably benefit. But . . . I hate to say this; I just don't like you! I just don't! There's something really unpleasant about you. I don't know. Maybe I can get my therapy and not deal with you." I felt flushed; at a loss for words, and started feeling I must really be unpleasant and I actually felt like running out of the room. The whole group was now looking at me. So, I chose to say exactly what I was feeling and thinking. After what seemed like a silent eternity, I turned to Tom and June and said "Thank you for helping to open this up." Then I asked Dana if he would say more, and that this time I would be prepared to listen to him fully, with a non-rebutting mind. He hesitantly essentially repeated what he'd said, and went on to add that he'd talked to his wife about his feelings and she too had urged him to talk about them in the group. He'd done so, but in the parking lot to Tom and June. I asked him if he wanted to continue talking, as he looked increasingly uncomfortable. He said no, he'd had enough for now. I then offered to replicate to him what he'd said. He nodded yes. I believe I repeated essentially accurately what he'd stated. He nodded, and said "Yup. You've got it." I felt some relief and said no more. The rest of the group talked about what had transpired for a while and then we went on to other matters. Later that day I discussed all this with a colleague, and found myself being aware of how stunned and hurt and angry I was at being the apparent object of such dislike. I never realized how seriously I needed to be liked! A flood of memories about past rejections, and a falling out with a friend came back as strong, immediate, and hurtful recollections. I also suddenly realized I had forgotten for a while that he was my patient, and that I was obliged to treat him! In the next group meeting, the session began as though nothing previously had transpired. I was inclined to go along, for a while. Dana gave me a quick glance and at the next break in the process I spoke, disclosing that I had consulted with a colleague and had come to realize how vulnerable I was to being intensely disliked "for no reason."

Also how I'd briefly forgotten my therapist role, and about my anger. I concluded that I was now back "on duty" in my role, but did not yet feel any closure on this. Dana now looked at me when I spoke, and then said he was sorry to have hurt my feelings, but, he added "this was supposed to be therapy, wasn't it?" I did not press Dana, but after about 3 weeks he began to examine his dislike of me.

It hinged largely on the reenactment of being sent away to boarding school at 14, against his and his mother's wishes. It was a "done deal" between his aloof father and the sadistic headmaster. Dana had fought against it with all his might, but lost. The referral to me and my group (school) brought it all back. This vignette illustrates my corrective emotional experience. My outside colleague and the group were skillful in not pushing me and in letting me work on this at my own pace. There was more subsequent work done with Dana, which I have not added to this account. Incidentally, my mention of subgroups stems from my agreement with Agazarian that subgroups are a major therapeutic entity. I have found useful Roy MacKenzie's developmental stages model (Engagement, Differentiation, Interpersonal Work, and Termination). Though there are endless boundaries and transient subgroupings going on, in effect, every minute, I have found MacKenzie's four developmental containers to be the most steady location for group members as they zigzag to termination. To quote MacKenzie (1997), "The phenomenon of group development provides the clinician with a powerful perspective in making sense of group events." I agree, and use them as a lens on process.

Another concept within interpersonal group psychotherapy is the group as a social microcosm. This refers to the inevitability with which group members will settle down and eventually display their public and private personas. It also refers to the unique entity, their group, eventually acquiring its own character, atmosphere, and configuration. Character defenses, being ego-syntonic, are soon visible. Ethnic, religious, and cross-cultural factors also emerge. In today's American society, every therapist should be trained and prepared to work with several major "minority" groups. The literature on group psychotherapy with various ethnic and national groups is slowly growing. Therapists who come from a national subgroup should likewise not get trapped into working only with their own people. Like the rest of us, they should cross-train. Expressiveness, nuances, and nonverbal communication vary a great deal, and can mask, distort, or conceal signs of disturbed interpersonal relationships.

Another core concept of the school of interpersonal group psychotherapy is the dialogic imperative of the "here and now." Historically, this treatment technique probably goes back to Fritz Perls and his Gestalt approach. It also was used widely in the 1960s, when "wild" therapy flourished, especially on the west coast. Its original purpose was to combine experiential process and cognate learning, along with high emotional involvement. The interpersonal group therapist's task is first to move members into a here-and-now frame, and then to initiate "process illumination," which means concurrently revealing one's analysis of or commentary on the group's here-and-now process—essentially "disclosure about the experience of disclosure."

It is obvious that no group or person can maintain a continuous and exclusive here-and-now focus. Inevitably, people will revert to past and outside material, including their current concerns about family, home, and work. The resistance to here-and-now can be intense and has cultural support. Many feel it to be a controlling gimmick, and oppose it strongly. I could not find in the relevant literature a discussion of when here-and-now is appropriate and when it is not. It can be experienced as assaultive and cultlike.

How does interpersonal treatment work? How do all the necessary and sufficient conditions and techniques combine to deliver effective change? The generic treatment design put forth by Yalom indicates that after patients have successfully adopted the here-and-now modality, the therapist systematically confronts each patient with the following process interrogatory, referred to as "illumination":

> Here is what your behavior is.
> Here's how your behavior makes others feel.
> Here's how your behavior influences the opinions others have of you.
> Here's how your behavior influences your opinion of yourself.
> Finally, the therapist and therapy ask "Are you satisfied with the world you have created?"

Interestingly, this sounds like an existential question, as well as the ultimate stage of a corrective emotional experience!

What is the operational self-concept of a trained interpersonal psychotherapist? In the Sullivanian mold, she is a participant-observer. She is also described as capable of being transparent with patients when it is appropriate, but not for self-enhancement. The therapist also spreads her empathy evenly to both "the attackers and the attacked," and considers herself a true equal of her patients. She rejects all causal talk set in the past, as this may bring on feelings of victimization and self-absolution. She keeps patients in the here-and-now flow of dialogue but allows them to move at their own rate. Her ultimate goal is the cognitive and affective integration of experience, leading to a level of maturity where people, despite being subjected to intense negativity, can forebear destroying each other. Interpersonal psychotherapy is practiced widely and in many variants. It is alive and well, and serves as a useful philosophical and conceptual base for many related approaches.

References

Agazarian, Y. M. (1992). Phases of development in system and systems-centered groups. In V. Schermer & M. Pines (Eds.), *The ring of fire*. London: Routledge.

Alexander, F., & French, R. M. (1946). *Psychoanalytic therapy*. Lincoln: University of Nebraska Press.

Beck, A. P., Dugo, J. M., Eng, A. M., & Lewis, C. M. (1986). The search for phases in group development. In L. S. Greenburg & W. M. Pinsof (Eds.), *The psychotherapeutic process*. New York: Guilford.

Bernard, H. S., & MacKenzie, K. R. (1994). *Basics of group psychotherapy*. New York: Guilford Press.

Evans, F. B. (1996). *Harry Stack Sullivan*. New York: Routledge.

Havens, L. (1987). *Approaches to the mind*. Cambridge: Harvard University Press.

Kivilighan, D. M., & Lilly, R. L. (1997). Developmental changes in group climate. *Group Dynamics, 1*(3), 208–221.

Klein, R. H., Bernard, H. S., & Singer, D. L. (Eds.). (1992). *Handbook of contemporary group psychotherapy.* Madison, CT: International University Press.

Leszcz, M. (1992). The interpersonal approach to group psychotherapy. *International Journal of Group Psychotherapy, 42* (1): 37–62.

MacKenzie, K. R. (1997). Clinical application of group developmental ideas. *Group Dynamics, 1*(3), 275–287.

McGrath, J. E. (1997). Small group research. *Group Dynamics, 1*, 7–27.

Nitsun, M. (1996). *The anti-group.* London: Routledge.

Pines, M. (1996). Malcolm Pines' reflections on Bridger, Main, Foulkes, & Bion–interviewed by Gary Winship. *Therapeutic Communities, 17* (2): 117–122.

Rogers, C. (1970). *Encounter groups.* New York: Harper & Row.

Rothke, S. (1986). The role of interpersonal feedback in group psychotherapy. *International Journal of Group Psychotherapy, 36*, 225–240.

Sullivan, H. S. (1954). *The psychiatric interview.* New York: Norton.

Winnicott, D. W. (1965). The theory of the parent-infant relationship. In *The maturational process and the facilitating environment.* New York: International Universities Press.

Yalom, I. D. (1993). *The theory and practice of group psychotherapy.* New York: Basic Books.

Yalom, I. D. (1995). *The theory and practice of group therapy* (4th ed.). New York: Basic Books.

Anxiety, Courage, and Healing

Maryetta Andrews-Sachs

> What heals people
> A closer look at insight
> Anxiety as opportunity
> The role of courage
> The transparent therapist

Healing

What heals people? The work of this Institute is to focus on how groups can heal people and how different approaches accomplish that task. We're all committed to the task of healing. But what do we really mean by "healing"? What makes a therapist a healer?

Irvin Yalom's words come to mind: "Effective psychotherapists, regardless of their stated psychotherapeutic orientation, share certain common attributes that include empathy, warmth, and acceptance . . . and are more alike than are effective and ineffective therapists of the same stated psychotherapeutic orientation" (1995).

Effective therapists also need courage and a high tolerance for anxiety. These components figure prominently in my approach to group therapy, and they mesh with my chosen therapeutic model: an approach that is interpersonal with a decidedly existential focus. I will discuss why I feel that the consideration of anxiety, courage, and therapist transparency, or openness, is so important and indeed, necessary to the healing process.

Virginia Satir (unpublished communication) once commented that wherever she went in the world she ran into the same eight people. In the interpersonal model all the information a therapist needs is in the room. Relationships with parents, siblings, peers—all significant others—will sooner or later be played out before the group's eyes.

What are the healing factors? I believe there are three: insight, catharsis, and reeducation, the reeducation being the most important. Now I will consider each of these.

Insight

Many colleagues—and patients—disagree when I say how unimportant insight is in the process of change. If insight worked so well, our patients (and potential patients) would head to the self-help section of the local book store, and we therapists would soon be out of work. Nevertheless, insight seems to be a starting point in the work and an important building block in the therapeutic relationship.

Something more must happen. Freud said, "Anyone who wants to make a living from the treatment of nervous patients must clearly be able to do something to help them" (1935). In fact, they must do more than facilitate insight. When a heart surgeon opens up a heart, he doesn't just say "Aha! There's the hole!" He fixes it. That doctor had to find that hole. The therapist must find the holes in the Self. But insight remains a very small part of what actually heals people.

Washington psychiatrist Herb Cohen has a business card he passes out as a joke. It reads: "Herb Cohen, Psychiatrist and Roofer: If your roof leaks, that's your business. If you want to fix it, that's my business." He believes in the therapist being fully present and active in the moment.

Rabbi Harold S. Kushner, author of *When Bad Things Happen to Good People*, also wrote *When Everything You Ever Wanted Isn't Enough*. Kushner studied the Book of Ecclesiastes in the Bible. Apparently, Ecclesiastes struggled to make his life work just like the rest of us, and Kushner (2002) summed up Ecclesiastes' findings with these three teachings:

1. Belong to people.

2. Accept pain as part of living.

3. Know that you make a difference.

That's an interesting measuring stick whether you're sitting with an individual or a group. They also match Yalom's analysis of curative factors in group psychotherapy rather well.

I think about what has healed me: a combination of love—and raising my tolerance for anxiety. In the preface to Ruthellen Josselson's book *The Space Between Us, Exploring the Dimensions of Human Relationships,* she writes, "What causes us embarrassment is to talk about love" (1995). When I think about love I think about accepting someone just as they are—a tall order indeed. Yet this sets the scene for personal growth. The therapist is then able to become the "encourager"—to lend courage so that the individual can dare to face what he needs to face.

In the Gospel of St. Thomas in the Dead Sea Scrolls Jesus is attributed as saying: "If you bring forth what is in you to bring forth, what you bring forth will save you; if you do not bring forth what is within you to bring forth, what you do not bring forth will destroy you."

I picture a therapy group as a place that creates an environment over time where it is safe to be vulnerable and allows that which needs to come forth to come forth. In our first weekend a member of the demonstration group said to another: "Even though you're vulnerable, I still see you as strong." I believe it takes courage and strength to be vulnerable because we live in a society where people interpret vulnerability as weakness.

Anxiety

Raising one's tolerance for normal anxiety, guilt, and despair is the cornerstone of real personality change. People need to learn from treatment that they have to do homework everyday, not just when they are meeting with their therapy group. Life provides many opportunities where every day a person can choose one path or another—and we human beings too often take the path of least resistance: no anxiety, thank you. It is unnatural for people to face anxiety; we have to be taught to do it.

We must ourselves learn and then teach our patients to do what is counterintuitive. For us to be the people we can be, we must find the courage to meet our anxiety, our guilt, our loneliness, and our depression head-on.

Ask yourself; what moments are the most anxiety-producing for you?

I cannot overstate the importance of this central point. Let me use myself and my development as a group therapist as an example. While in college I had the opportunity to attend a weekend at the University of Chicago entitled "Conversations with Paul Tillich." I sat at the knee of one of the great thinkers of the 20th century. Yet I remember nothing he said. I was too anxious, too bound-up, on "automatic pilot" as a human being. Rollo May, writing about the difference between anxiety and fear, said: "The basic difference is that anxiety strikes at the central core of one's self-esteem and sense of value as a self. Anxiety is, therefore, an important aspect of the experience of self as a being. Fear, in contrast, is a threat to the periphery of one's existence, blots out his sense of time, dulls his memory of the past, and erases the future. These effects are the most compelling demonstration and proof that anxiety attacks the very center of one's being" (1992).

My colleague, George Saiger (1996), has written that Hugh Mullen didn't much like Yalom's book, *Existential Psychotherapy*. Hugh's point was that "the crux of the matter was that the therapist, not the therapy, be existentially there." In other words, if we cannot bear the anxiety of the material evoked during a session, it doesn't matter how well we intellectually understand the material. I believe, on the other hand, Yalom's work is one book every therapist should read. But just as Tillich was once lost on me, so would Yalom's book have been lost on me without the long years of effort I needed to raise my very low tolerance for anxiety. Years ago, I would have read it, believed it to be very wise, but it would not have touched me.

In my early years as a therapist, I attended many conferences and encounter groups. I went to Esalen, got Rolfed, spent time in the Catskills with Baba Muktanunda. I went through EST, attended several AK Rice Institutes. I did all this in addition to individual therapy for eons.

In long-term group psychotherapy I had to finally wrestle my Self to the ground. I was like a person frozen in place unable to access my thoughts or feelings. The computer screen in my head was blank. Only by risking every time, and thereby raising my tolerance for anxiety, did I slowly chip away my armor and begin to discover my true Self.

When I was appointed chair of this weekend, I felt an old familiar terror. I thought, *Oh my God, I'll be exposed as a fraud. I don't know enough. Only white males can do this. I've spent the last 13 years reading children's books.* I searched around and found multiple terrific reasons not to chair this weekend. But then I asked myself the basic question I am always asking others: Am I making this decision from a position of strength or weakness? Can I not draw on 25 years of experience in groups—as a therapist, a supervisee, a supervisor, and as a patient?

I began to realize what a fraud I would be if I sat in my office and told others to see anxiety as opportunity and face it—and then didn't myself. Experience has taught me that when we face something we're afraid of, there's something inside us that says, "Oh, I did it! I survived!" Our self-esteem and self-respect go up. If we shrink from it, and don't find the courage to face it, our self-esteem and self-respect shrink.

People who come to see us must be helped to see exactly where they need to raise their tolerance for anxiety, where they are avoiding it, and how their "presenting problem" is connected to having too low a tolerance. Once they have a relationship with the therapist, and when the patient can tolerate the anxiety evoked in a group, a group is the best place to do this work.

Courage

Do you talk to your patients about courage? I often think of Paul Tillich's (1952) seminal work *The Courage to Be*. Tillich writes about each of us having the courage to be fully alive, *in spite of* our anxiety. He assumes we are anxious, this being part of the human condition. Furthermore, he separates "the courage to be" into two parts—the courage to be oneself—and the courage to be a part, meaning a participant in a relationship, a family, a community. How different the world would look if we each had the courage to be both autonomous and intimate.

We readily recognize the courage it takes for most people to seek treatment. When they come to us, we have the opportunity to encourage them to develop attitudes about life that will stay with them long after treatment ends.

Rollo May wrote a wonderful book, *Paulus: Tillich as Spiritual Teacher.* It is the story of May's 30-year relationship with Tillich, his mentor and friend. May describes Tillich as someone very private; and yet his students, friends, and colleagues always knew what Tillich was feeling. If he was embarrassed or upset or excited—they knew. Tillich embodied the belief that having the courage to be meant being whomever one really is at that moment. May writes the following:

> The Self is the stronger the more non-being* it can take into itself. Thus if we can accept *normal* anxiety and guilt, if we can live with our anger, we become the stronger; but we also find, as in the psychotherapeutic confrontation of anger, that feelings of love also increase. The anxiety turns out not to be so unbearable after all, and our pretense in trying to repress it simply a way of putting off our experience of life.

Transparency

Now I will try to be more courageous and talk about the role of transparency—openness—in group therapy and more about how I work. In the theory of the interpersonal model, the therapist's role is that of a participant-observer, a concept developed by Harry Stack Sullivan (1940). What does this mean? How far can one go in being open about oneself?

Yalom talks of "judicious disclosure." Many therapists believe telling a patient something about oneself is the equivalent of committing a deadly sin. But I believe there is a lot of stealth transparence that occurs with no one willing to admit it.

For example, I was visiting with a friend whom I had not seen for sometime, and I learned she was in therapy with my first supervisor. I vividly recall this supervisor's very strong dictum against any kind of transparency and so I was amazed when my friend described the change that had occurred in her therapy after her therapist had her first baby—at a late age. This therapist continued to hold to her position of revealing little about herself, but readily talked about her little girl, showed pictures, and described weekly incidents.

Did this therapist think she wasn't revealing something about herself? Did the revelations harm the therapy in my friend's eyes? Actually my friend felt the disclosures had enhanced it, brought them closer, opened up new areas for exploration of mother-daughter relationships, including their relationship. On the other hand, I've been taken aback when certain therapists have gone through incredibly powerful experiences in their own lives and said nothing.

But how do we measure whether sharing something is self-indulgent? Or, are we being self-protective and missing an opportunity to be in the moment with that person or group? Is it possible that we make a virtue of necessity by landing hard and fast on one position about this? We ask our patients to risk being vulnerable,

---

* Non-being—anxiety, guilt, fear, loneliness, and depression.

authentic, and courageous. Why not model this at judicious moments? Is not our failure to do this a failure to act courageously? Do we not infantilize patients by asking them to completely reveal themselves while we reveal nothing?

Now let me be clear. Regardless of orientation, a good therapist pays very close attention to his own emotional life and uses himself as a diagnostic tool. So I am talking about sharing other personal material with a patient or group, such as a dream, an incident with a "significant other," a memory, or where one is going on vacation.

I am a transparent therapist and proud of it. This is not an easy road. I struggle every hour with many considerations and "rules of thumb" in my head. Here are some of them.

The Sicker the Patient, the Tighter the Boundaries

For example, with borderline patients, I give no personal information about myself other than the immediate emotional material relevant to our relationship. However, I have found that as years pass, it is evidence of great change in the patient when more personal material can be brought in and managed. I have seen one woman for 22 years. In the early years she had to be hospitalized when I went on vacation. She was unable to tolerate evidence that I had a life outside of our relationship. These days, when she's not too busy to get in for an appointment, we can discuss anything from her life or mine.

Omission Rather Than Commission

When in doubt I share nothing. When uncertain of why I might be tempted to share something I weigh several things first. One big consideration is *timing*. Early in the treatment the patient often needs to see us as powerful and able to help them. They may feel abandoned and helpless if we reveal our own vulnerabilities too soon. They may need a certain picture of us in place for some time.

If we share some of our own vulnerabilities too soon some patients may feel they have to take care of us. They may experience us as needy and think we are asking them for help rather than vice versa.

Feelings of jealousy may be evoked in patients by our providing certain material about our lives. Also the exploration of fantasies and other feelings about the therapist is such a rich area of our work and not to be ignored. But in the interest of developing more authentic relationships, I would opt for exploring the patient's fantasies first—and then, depending on the stage of treatment, bring in the reality.

Look at This Issue From a Systems Point of View

The therapist might consider whether she is allowing herself to be seduced by the group in order to avoid more anxiety-producing work. As much as I love groups and believe in their tremendous therapeutic value, I'm always aware of this down-side: that *a mutual defense pact* can unconsciously be struck among members of the group—including me—to avoid anxiety. "You don't mention that subject and I won't bring up that issue between you and Bill," etc.

Am I Being Self-Indulgent?

To have someone fascinated with you is very seductive. It is also a terrific way to help the patient avoid the anxiety of dealing with himself or for the therapist to avoid difficult issues in the treatment.

In my experience, "judicious disclosure" can be another building block in the therapeutic alliance. But it must be used wisely. Many people enter treatment with some agenda of their own in the form of presenting symptoms. Chatting endlessly about the therapist's life usually doesn't top the patient's list. Don't you think that would create boredom and resentment after awhile? Also the real work of therapy could be avoided by all parties concerned, the patient could terminate believing they had therapy, and they might never know otherwise.

Furthermore, I believe that not sharing some real material can be infantilizing to the patient. Do we believe patients can't tolerate or assimilate information about where we're going on vacation? Do we not unconsciously feed patients illusions that if they're really good we might tell them whether we have children or struggle ourselves? Are we not possibly more credible when we get to what is unknowable in life, or what only they can answer for themselves, if we've been open about what we do and don't know? The ultimate purpose of the psychoanalytic posture of "nondisclosure" or abstinence is to force the patient from the pleasure principle to the reality principle. Don't we do that more effectively by letting patients know that we do care and as much as we would like to, can't do for them what they must do for themselves?

References

Freud, S. (1935). *An autobiographical study*. London: Hogarth Press.

Josselson, R. (1995). *The space between us: Exploring the dimensions of human relationships*. Thousand Oaks, CA: Sage Publications.

Kushner, H. (2002).*When all you've ever wanted isn't enough: The search for a life that matters*. New York: Fireside Press.

May, R. (1992). *Paulus: Tillich as spiritual teacher*. Peter Smith.

Mullen, H., & Sangiuliano, I. (1964). *The therapist's contribution to the treatment process: His person, transactions and treatment methods*. Springfield, IL: Charles C. Thomas.

Saiger, G. (1996). Some thoughts on the Existential Lens in Group Therapy. *Group, 20* (2).

Sullivan, H. (1940). Conceptions of modern psychiatry: The first Wiliam Alanson White Memorial Lecture. *Psychiatry, 3*(1).

Tillich, P. (1952). *The courage to be*. New Haven: Yale University Press.

Yalom, I.D. (1995). *The theory and practice of group psychotherapy* (4th ed.). New York: Basic Books.

The Interpersonal Approach
to Group Psychotherapy

Molyn Leszcz

Effective psychotherapists, regardless of their stated psychotherapeutic orientation, share certain common attributes that include empathy, warmth, and acceptance (Luborsky, Crits-Christoph, Mintz, & Averbach, 1988) and are more alike than are effective and ineffective therapists of the same stated psychotherapeutic orientation (Yalom, 1985). At the same time, the therapist's orientation and conceptualization of what are the mutative elements in group psychotherapy will invariably shape therapeutic interventions and the therapist functions assumed within the group. Accordingly, this article will focus on the interpersonal model of group psychotherapy and the interpersonal interactions within the group as the nucleus of change, growth, and improvement, a model best articulated by Yalom (1985). Beginning with the essential contributions of Harry Stack Sullivan (1953) to interpersonal theory and moving forward to include the contributions of contemporary theoreticians and clinicians (Kiesler & Anchin, 1982; Safran & Segal, 1990; Strupp & Binder, 1984), certain fundamental principles emerge.

Each individual has a central human drive for interpersonal attachment and the maintenance of self-worth within interpersonal terms. Personality is a relatively enduring pattern of recurrent interpersonal transactions and interactions, and each person's self system is essentially interpersonal in that it is composed of reflected appraisals of significant others (Sullivan, 1953). The developing individual embraces those parts of the self that are valued by his or her significant others, and lead to maintenance of attachment, and disavows through the mechanism of selective inattention those parts of the self or the environment that create anxiety by threatening self-worth and attachment. Relatively enduring personality traits develop consequently (Merman, Weissman, Rounsaville, & Chevron, 1984). A child's early sense of having his or her emotional experiences matched by those of significant others, the process of affect attunement (Safran & Segal, 1990), is one of the major mechanisms that convey to the individual how he or she is appraised by others and confirms that his or her emotional experience is a human and shareable one. Mismatch induces in the child the feeling that his or her experience is not acceptable or shareable and that it needs to be concealed with the consequent constriction of the self and interpersonal interactions. Repair is possible if the secondary emotional reactions—for example, anger masking sadness—are responded to appropriately, in a way that allows the child's original feeling to be addressed. If not, then initial constriction may lead to an ever-increasing sense of restriction in access to the self and others. Effective affect attunement leads to a process of repair of inevitable disappointments, and the child developing a sense of relationships carrying warranties rather than guarantees, resulting in greater willingness to explore a broad range of engaging behaviors.

Psychological disturbance is a consequence of disturbed interpersonal relationships and is manifested in disturbed interpersonal communication and interaction. This disturbance can be seen in verbal, paraverbal, and nonverbal methods of communication, often unconscious to the individual. These reflect parataxic distortions—rigid, characteristic generalizations of past relationships crystallized by memory and symbolization—that are transferred on to contemporary relationships (Sullivan, 1953). A series of interpersonal transactions follow in which an initial distortion-based communication shapes and elicits a predictable complementary interpersonal response, resulting potentially in an interpersonal recapitulation or vicious circle of reverberating transactions. The traditional idea of linear causality is supplanted by one of circular causality (Kiesler & Anchin, 1982). For example, a person who has come to anticipate interpersonal rejection, believing the cause of rejection is his or her expression of feelings or desires, may interact in a very bland, unidimensional, unengaged mode. Revealing nothing of himself or herself that is real or authentic will cause relationships to wither, thereby confirming the initial belief, and the correctness of the anticipated rejection. Clearly this will have a deleterious effect on self-worth and self-esteem, resulting in a further narrowing of expressions of the self. Each individual thereby initiates the authoring of his or her own interpersonal environment by the dual process of maladaptive construal of the environment and subsequent maladaptive behaviors (Strupp & Binder, 1984). The attempted solution becomes the problem.

In related fashion, Safran and Segal (1990) have introduced the concept of the interpersonal schema—a generic core cognitive structure based on early interpersonal experiences that contains information relevant to the maintenance of interpersonal relatedness. The schema integrates and shapes both one's processing of cognitive and affective information and one's subsequent implementation of actions. It encompasses one's expectations, contingencies, goals, and strategies. An individual may have several interrelated interpersonal schemas. They suggest that all cognitive structures are subordinate to the goal of maintenance of interpersonal connection—the biologically driven need for attachment.

A central concept of interpersonal group psychotherapy is that the focus of clinical study is the phenomenology and process of the patient–therapist relationship, which, if properly scrutinized, leads to illumination of the parataxic distortions and maladaptive interpersonal patterns. The patient–therapist relationship is the microscopic here-and-now "part" that reflects the "whole" of the patient's macroscopic world. The therapist actively examines his or her reactions to the patient, using this information to deepen the understanding of the patient's interpersonal core. The therapist is both participant and observer. Hence transference and countertransference are integrally linked and addressed by both the patient and the therapist in collaboration. Transference is relationship driven and the patient's reactions are functions of his or her interpersonal schema and the interpersonal tints in his or her environment, as they are subjectively perceived. Contemporary relationships are perceived in old, often outmoded models. Non-schema-compatible stimuli, either internal or external, are ignored by virtue of the use of selective inattention. Similarly, countertransference is a function of the therapist's interpersonal predispositions and the unavoidable reactions evoked by the patient's interpersonal communications, the relative contribution of which falls on the therapist to ascertain.

The therapist's lack of attention to the interpersonal process ensures maintenance of the vicious circle. It is impossible not to get "hooked" (Kiesler & Anchin, 1982) by the patient consciously or unconsciously; deed, the hooking process is essential to the therapy. The challenge for the therapist is to get unhooked in order to process, with the patient, the patient's interactional style: what it evoked in and how it affected the therapist. To illustrate, a patient like the one described in the earlier example might readily hook the therapist into experiencing him or her as bland, perhaps even boring. Compliance and lack of emotions might go unchallenged in the therapy and might even be unnoticed by the therapist. Accordingly, little attention may be paid to the range of ways in which the patient conceals genuine expressions of the self and obstructs any real engagement with the therapist. Intellectual insight is only partially corrective. What is required is the penitential disconfirmation within the therapeutic relationship of the client's fundamental maladaptive conceptualizations of the self in relationship to the interpersonal environment and the patient's recognition of his or her related contributions.

The "hooking–unhooking" process is a therapeutic bridge to the therapist's empathic awareness of the patient's interpersonal schema allowing the therapist to respond in a concordant and attuned mode … in a complementary and circular mode. The patient is invited to deepen the phenomenological exploration of the contemporary relationship in collaboration with the therapist, elaborating affects, attitudes, and beliefs. In fact, Weiss and Sampson's (1986) analysis of process in psychotherapy supports their contention that the patient's central objective therapy is to obtain evidence that his or her core pathogenic belief in the maintenance of attachments will be disconfirmed. This disconfirmation accrues both from insight and the experiential elements of the treatment relationship, and results in the patient feeling greater safety about further disclosure and engagement.

In order to challenge the patient's core interpersonal concepts and constructs, the therapeutic encounter must be sufficiently emotionally alive to the patient. Hence, experience-near processing of the contemporary treatment relationship is superior to experience-far processing of past or external relationships. A stable relationship and intact therapeutic alliance are prerequisites both to the illumination and to the processing aspects of therapy, mitigating against the patient's experiencing feedback as critical, demeaning, and inadvertently schema confirming. The feedback to the patient is presented in a collaborative mode, examined mutually rather than dictated unilaterally by the therapist. The processing leads to an ever-evolving hypothesis of the individual's interpersonal schema. Close scrutiny of the patient–therapist interaction may reveal certain prototypical points—interpersonal markers—that are iceberg tips of deeper interpersonal beliefs and attitudes (Safran & Segal, 1990). These markers are signs within the therapeutic relationship of some shift in relatedness or affective experience, both verbal and nonverbal. For example, continuing from the earlier example, such a marker might be the patient withdrawing or turning more quiet following a tentative expression of a feeling, or wish, in the therapy. If this shift can be detected and illuminated, it provides a very vital opportunity to deepen the exploration of the patient's view of his or her self and interpersonal world. These are red flags for further phenomenological exploration, the starting point always being the patient's affective experience.

In the actual flow of the therapy, effective disconfirmation of interpersonal schemas or pathogenic beliefs (Weiss & Sampson et al., 1986) will be reflected in the patient's diminished anxiety, deeper elaboration of schema-related material, both contemporary and historical, and increased self-awareness. Effective disconfirmation results in a broadening of the individual's interpersonal repertoire and choices, fuller emotional participation in interactions, and a shift from subjective perceptions to consensually validated and objective perceptions. Changes are noted first in the therapeutic setting and later in the patient's everyday life. It follows that the therapist needs to have the broadest possible range of understanding of interpersonal communications and their significance. It is accordingly an approach that has as its central focus the maintenance of the individual's self-esteem and interpersonal connections.

Although this approach emphasizes the contemporary relationship, there is much relevance in exploration of the past, particularly when historical material is brought forward by the patient spontaneously, following disconfirmation and challenging of his or her interpersonal schema. Historical reconstruction may help the patient make sense of patterns or decrease a sense of shame or guilt over dysfunctional behaviors by examining what has given rise to them. Furthermore, understanding the past can stimulate feelings of greater faith about the capacity for change. However, adherence to the past can be an escape from more intimate, high-risk exposure in the contemporary situation. Hence a key principle in processing historical information is its linkage to the here-and-now, and how alive the patient is emotionally, in the exploration.

Grunebaum and Solomon's (1987) comprehensive review of the development of peer relatedness argues strongly for the indivisibility of the sense of self and peer relationships. They believe that peer relationships ultimately supplant the primary relationship with the parents, providing new opportunities for self-exploration and self-correction. If we accept these principles about interpersonal relationships and the importance of the peer group then we can develop a model of group therapy that emphasizes peer relatedness, the correction of interpersonal distortions, and disconfirmation of maladaptive interpersonal schemas, and teaches members interpersonal skills to break maladaptive interpersonal recapitulations. How the therapist brings this to life will be elaborated in the next section, following a brief review of research confirming these concepts.

Research Findings

The therapeutic mechanism of interpersonal learning is highly valued across virtually all studies of therapeutic factors in group therapy and is particularly valued by successfully treated patients (Yalom, 1985). This is certainly true in ambulatory settings, but there is evidence that when groups are structured to emphasize interpersonal learning opportunities, even in acute care inpatient environments, this factor is highly valued (Leszcz, Yalom, & Norden, 1985). Weiner (1974) challenged the importance of dynamic insight relative to genetic insight but found that despite his initial hypothesis that genetic insight would be more highly valued by his patients, discovered that dynamic, interpersonal insight was the more highly valued. In a more recent study, Flowers and Booraem (1990) found that in comparing psychoanalytic therapists and cognitive behavioral therapists the interventions that were most linked to positive outcome were here-and-now dynamic interpersonal interventions that illuminated patterns and effects of behavior. Interestingly, both types of therapists used psychodynamic and cognitive-behavioral interventions. Jargonistic interpretations of motivation and historical causality were less highly valued and were particularly of no value if they were negatively worded or carried a blaming tone. It is noteworthy that co-patients were often more effective than were the therapists in making genetic linkages, because of their utilization of less complex wordings.

Bloch and Crouch (1985) in their review of therapeutic factors echo the work of Strupp and Binder (1984) in their conclusion that insight is only useful if it is accepted by the patient and if it registers. The closer the therapist stays to consensually validated, here-and-now information, the harder it is for the patient to refute it. The here-and-now has inherent face validity, while interpretations aimed at genetic reconstruction may convey to patients a sense of distance. It appears easier to access a patient's motivation after pattern and impact are elucidated, rather than the converse.

Models of group therapy that emphasize rigid interpretation of a central group-as-a-whole transference to the leader, devaluing peer transferences as mutative, have outcomes no better than nontreatment. Furthermore, strict group therapist abstinence from interaction evokes patient complaints about insufficient human and interpersonal engagement (Malan, Balfour, Hood, & Shooter, 1976). Shifts in orientation from group-centered, leader-centered, interpretive modes to a more peer interactional model has been associated with increased therapist and patient satisfaction with significant improvement in patient acceptance of group psychotherapy (Azim & Joyce, 1986).

Interpersonal Group Psychotherapy

Having discussed the critical importance of interpersonal relationships as a window through which the therapist is best able to access the internal world of the patients in the group I will try to identify the key ingredients of the interpersonal psychotherapy group. Central elements include group cohesion; the group providing a corrective emotional experience; the group operating as a social microcosm; the essential role of feedback in interpersonal learning; and the overarching principle of working in the here-and-now (Yalom, 1985).

Cohesion and Group Process

Although the interpersonal approach to group therapy emphasizes interpersonal learning it is important to note that all other traditional group therapeutic factors (Moth & Crouch, 1985; Yalom, 1985) are also operative. In fact, no therapeutic factor stands apart from an interpersonal context. However, opportunities for interpersonal learning will arise only if the therapist establishes that as a priority. The first step involves the establishment and maintenance of a cohesive group. Cohesion operates as a therapeutic factor in that feelings of acceptance and belonging may be mutative and corrective for some individuals, but even more importantly cohesion serves as a met therapeutic factor, in that it facilitates expression of all the other therapeutic factors. Group cohesion is parallel to the therapeutic alliance in individual psychotherapy. In the same way that a stable therapeutic alliance in individual therapy is linked to positive outcome (Luborsky et al., 1988; Safran & Segal, 1990), group cohesion is similarly related to factors that contribute to positive outcome. In addition to being highly valued by successful patients, group cohesion has been linked to increased task adherence; increased attendance and diminished dropouts; increased self-disclosure; and increased conflict resolution with a greater level of tolerance for expressed hostility (Yalom, 1985). Individuals within cohesive groups are more self-accepting and open to the influence of others (Yalom, 1985). In order for patients to be able to bring themselves honestly and fully to the group they must trust that the group is durable, present, and can tolerate and contain their emotional expression without fragmentation or flight. In this regard it functions as a holding environment (Modell, 1976). Hence overstimulation of affect beyond the capacity of the individual or the group as a whole should be avoided in the early phases of group development. Ruptures in the feeling of connectedness to the group occur regularly, in particular with characterologically difficult patients, and need to be examined and repaired each time within the context of the subjective experience of the event that induced the rupture (Leszcz, 1989).

An important point of demarcation of this model from group-centered approaches is the idea that, in this model, the therapist takes active responsibility as a facilitator to stimulate and invite cohesive engagement between members of the group. Patients turning to one another is not necessarily a flight or displacement from an unreachable, noninteractive therapist, but rather it is the pursuit of positive peer relationships, promoted by initial feelings of alikeness and a wish for acceptance. Peer relationships and peer transference are a primary phenomenon of the group's life. Accordingly, the therapist helps the group members successfully work through the early-phase fears of not being accepted and not belonging, recognizing the associated fear of loss of self through overinvolvement. These fears and apprehensions are viewed as developmentally appropriate and expectable, and at the same time members are invited to examine how they can begin to make the group feel safer for themselves.

From the outset the therapist establishes norms of valuing the group, of responsible self-disclosure, and of turning the attention of the group back onto itself, examining the interpersonal interactions between and amongst its members, in the here and now. The leader attempts to demystify his or her power and reflect back to the group the capacity to help one another and the therapeutic efficacy they each have with one another. Patients are invited to offer their subjective experiences of what is occurring within the group and at the same time to elicit feedback to begin the process of interpersonal exploration. Interpersonal feedback elicited at this point may focus more on feelings of attraction and acceptance to avoid stimulation of hostility before the group has confidence in its ability to tolerate strong negative emotions. Although members of the group will all work at their own pace, it is appropriate to try and balance the level of self-disclosure within the group such that no one patient deviates excessively from the group by virtue of monopolization or reticence. These patient postures reflect an underlying interpersonal process, and it is useful to begin exploration of the experience of silence, or of excessive verbalization, both for the individual and for others.

Notwithstanding emphasis on the interpersonal interactions, particularly in the group's early life, group developmental processes may affect the group as a whole in ways that contribute to the emergence of group-centered tensions about dependency, acceptance, power, and control being expressed by particular individuals, as scapegoats or monopolizers. The interpersonally oriented group therapist first addresses the group-centered process of resistance, which obstructs genuine interpersonal engagement, and then focuses on the interpersonal world of the group members, in contrast to other models that view the group process as primary and interaction as secondary (Kibel & Stein, 1981).

Group-as-a-whole processes that interfere with interpersonal engagement often reflect group-centered anxiety about the stability, integrity, or therapeutic capacity of the group, or the establishment of antitherapeutic group norms, and are likely to be reflected in group themes or particular group-as-whole postures.

As Bion (1961) described, participation in an unstructured group is quite regressive, reflecting anxieties about attachment and acceptance. The abstinent, non-responsive therapist heightens this regression, in order to illuminate individual's reactions to these forces, while the facilitative, interactive therapist diminishes it. The group therapist offers preparation, through both support and information to incoming group members, to mitigate the undue anxiety that invariably is present in the beginning phases of a group. The therapist tries to reduce these tensions by anticipating them.

Clinical Illustration
One session before two new members replaced senior members who had recently terminated the group, the group members began the session with a cascade of expressions of anxiety. They elaborated a highly suspicious, challenging stance. The manifest content centered around one of the members of the group, Joe, who had at the end of the last session seen someone he believed to be one of the group's observers going to the washroom with a smirk on his face. This enraged Joe, who felt he was providing entertainment for the observers and that be was at their mercy. He feared that he could run into an observer in a social situation and have the humiliating and vulnerable experience of knowing nothing about the other person and yet having the other person know every kind of intimate detail about him. Other people in the group echoed his sentiments and complained about the intrusiveness of observers and the power indiscreet observers had to do harm to the members of the group. Although the group had been ongoing, and each member in the group consented to the observation as part of a teaching hospital mandate, members of the group began to agitate for change: eliminating observers, bringing the observers into the room so that they would not be faceless figures, or, as a last resort, drawing the curtains so that the group members could be heard but not seen.

The power of the group process was quite profound and the therapist found himself beginning to be swayed, wondering if there had been some breach of discretion or confidentiality. In the midst of rising antagonism and anxiety, the therapist suggested that the acute sense of tension, suspicion, and vulnerability may have much less to do with who was watching the group from behind the mirror than with who was going to be entering the group imminently and watching from in front of the mirror. The loss of two valued members and the entry of two "strangers" no doubt induced anxiety about the group's ability to function effectively and with safety. Could the integrity and boundaries of the group be maintained? The therapist added that more relevant than what people outside of the group thought was what the people inside the group thought of one another at this particular moment. What apprehensions did they have about information they provided to one another that might be used destructively? Who appeared safe? Who appeared to be threatening to them right now in the group?

These kinds of threats to group integrity occur regularly and predictably at boundary-points in the group's life. These may include therapist's absences, exit or entry of members to the group, or the presence of strong dysphoric or negative affects that threaten the group members' confidence in the group's functioning as a holding environment. These logjams, either silent and stagnant or loud and antagonistic, need to be worked through before further work can proceed at the level of members' interpersonal issues.

Recognizing the fundamental importance of interpersonal relationships to the individuals in the group, and the therapist's perspective that it is through these interpersonal interactions that each person's characteristic view of self and of the interpersonal world is illuminated, it becomes essential for the therapist to shape the group to facilitate its capacity to maximize members' interpersonal engagement in the here-and-now. It is both the richest aspect of group therapy and yet for many therapists and patients the most unnatural and difficult (Zaslav, 1988). At the outset, patients will not be able to turn their attention to the interpersonal transactions without guidance or direction. They will be much more focused on the then-and-there, telling their story, often seeking relief rather than growth. Many patients will find it initially dissonant to consider that their identified difficulties can be accessed via the study of interpersonal transactions. Pregroup preparation is invaluable in easing patients' entry into the group, reducing obstructive anxiety, increasing attendance and task adherence, and working in the here-and-now (Yalom, 1985). The assessment interviews themselves can begin the educative process of reforming the patients' concerns into interpersonal terms. A detailed history of significant relationships, interactional patterns, and transactions emphasizes this point to the patient, and provides the therapist with useful interpersonal schema-relevant material.

Corrective Emotional Experience
Illumination of interpersonal difficulty is insufficient and may even be assaultive if repair is not possible. Horner (1975) comments on the importance of identifying the subjective experience that lies beneath the manifest interpersonal defense, to safeguard against the patient experiencing feedback as a narcissistic attack. This is particularly relevant for patients whose interpersonal defenses manifest themselves in haughtiness, devaluing of others, and relative disregard of the internal experiences of their co-members, thereby inviting hostile counteractions. The process of repair is not just insight; it must contain an experiential component. Hence, Yalom (1985) extended Alexander and French's (1946) idea of treatment offering a corrective emotional experience to the group therapy setting.

By virtue of their recapitulative interpersonal cycles, patients unwittingly evoke the interactions that they fear the most, and the group environment provides enormous opportunity for the emergence of characteristic reactions to powerful interpersonal issues such as intimacy, conflict, power, and belonging. The phenomenon of interpersonal recapitulation may be conceptualized in a variety of ways. It may be a learned behavior, repeated as a result of social learning and relative blindness to alternative approaches, hooking complementary, circular responses (Kiesler & Anchin, 1982). Alternatively it may be an unconsciously determined attempt on the individual's part to test the significant other, hoping that the significant other will disconfirm a fundamental belief about the self and the interpersonal world (Weiss & Sampson et al., 1981). Or the psychoanalytic concept of projective identification (Horvitz, 1983) may be useful. An interpersonal transaction is created by the use of this unconscious defense, as the subject projects an unacceptable part of the self into the significant other. The projection is incomplete, however, and the subject remains identified with the projected components and seeks actively to keep the disavowed parts of self out of himself or herself and contained within the object. By turning the passive into the active, often through unconscious identification with the original perpetrator of emotional injury, the subject masters feelings of helplessness, threats of abandonment, or feelings of worthlessness by projecting and containing these feelings within the object. The projector further attempts to control the behavior of the object on line with these projected elements. If the object responds in complementary and retaliatory fashion, and attacks, devalues, or rejects the projector, the interpersonal recapitulation continues. If, however, the object is able to respond in a concordant fashion using internal experience to increase empathic understanding of the subject, he or she is able to respond in a way that detoxifies the original fear and begins a process of repair, which is, ultimately, the unconscious hope of the projector. Accordingly, as in the hooking–unhooking sequence, the therapist's recognition and processing of his or her own reactions to the patient are essential.

In individual psychotherapy the therapist need be concerned primarily with his or her own reaction or countertransference to the patient's transference. In the group not only will the therapist need to contend with this working through process, the therapist must also be concerned with the reaction of other members of the group who are objects of projection. The therapist may need to model and set group norms such that all group members can ultimately move toward a position of supporting exploration, growth, and the process of working through, thereby providing restitution and disconfirmation, without biting at the interpersonal bait. A mature, well-functioning group will readily engage in both the initial stimulation of affect and disclosure, and the subsequent cognitive integration of the experience, if the therapist is able to demonstrate the rationale for this model of evocation and processing.

Social Microcosm
Ultimately, as initial anxiety and social niceties diminish, the group becomes a social microcosm and interpersonal laboratory in which members behave and interact, as they typically do in their outside world reproducing their characteristic maladaptive interpersonal styles. In vivo, here-and-now behavior becomes a much more reliable and valid focus of the therapy rather than the patients' reportage. There is a significant reduction of potential treatment blind spots that could be untouched within the individual setting either because the individual setting does not catalyze it; it is ego-syntonic to the individual and hence outside of that report; it is a mutual, synchronous blind spot of attitude or behavior shared by

the patient and therapist; or, because so much interpersonal communication is not verbal, it is beyond the individual's awareness to report (Bellak, 1980). The patient's entire composite behavior is open to scrutiny within the group including verbal, nonverbal, and paraverbal behaviors such as nuance, tone, and inflection. A facial expression may be worth a thousand words. The multiplicity of relationship opportunities in the group further provides a comprehensive elaboration of each individual's interpersonal schemas in an irrefutable, experience-near fashion. Ormont (1988) comments on the necessity of patients bringing themselves to the group in their full and characteristic fashion. Hence, the patient who resists engagement, elaborates a range of defenses against intimacy, or challenges the group's working is indeed much more actively involved in the group than is the compliant patient, who quietly keeps out of the group's life. In the latter situation, the dynamic of compliance or emotional surrender to the object becomes a here-and-now behavior that needs to be addressed in and of itself.

The Here-and-Now
Certainly the past has importance, and intercurrent issues emerge from members of the group that need to be addressed within the group as part of the integrity of the individual's experience. However, in each and every instance, the objective within this model is to evaluate, within the process, what the here-and-now ramifications are of the content of patient's report and the feedback it receives. Although the group members may be more naturally inclined to pursue vertical disclosure soliciting facts about external events, albeit presented in one-sided fashion by the subject, the group therapist is interested not only in this vertical disclosure but also the horizontal disclosure about the experience of disclosure. What analogue in the here and now has been touched upon at this particular moment? What is the experience of self-disclosure? What more can the patient say about what he or she is feeling at this moment? What made it possible for the patient to present this information today? How is he or she experiencing the group's reaction? What were the expectations and fears? Who was expected to be responsive? Who was expected to be critical? Can the patient examine rather than remain stuck within these assumptions? Hence content is inseparable from process, as lyrics are from a song's melody.

Processing the group in this fashion ensures that the group remains centripetally directed. All members feel close to the action as they begin to recognize that disclosure of their subjective experiences and feedback is essential. Patients will not arrive naturally at the process of giving feedback. The model set by the therapist through pregroup orientation, therapeutic transparency, and norm setting will shape the in-group process by which feedback is given. By emphasizing an ongoing reframing from the general to the specific, from the impersonal to the personal, and from the personal to the interpersonal, the therapist sets the stage for the therapeutic mechanism of interpersonal learning. Feedback appears to be most useful under the following conditions: it is clear and immediate, reflecting the here and now; it is communicated simply and without jargon; it contains an emotional component on the part of the sender of feedback and conveys some message about the relationship between the sender and the receiver of the feed- back; and the sender takes some risk in disclosing this communication. It is best presented in a nonpejorative and nonjudgmental fashion that leaves the receiver free to assess his or her own responsibility for making relationships better or worse (Rothke, 1986). Feedback is always a transaction that informs about both parties. The questioner both stakes disclosures about himself or herself and reac- tions to others.

Yalom (1985) has comprehensively articulated these factors into a model of group psychotherapy in which affective disclosure, by the individual and other members' feedback, is the key generator that is then processed and integrated cognitively, via a self-reflection loop. Groups that emphasize either affective stimulation and catharsis, or cognitive integration at the expense of the other, are limited in their effectiveness. A typical, effective sequence includes several steps: (1) The individual manifests a characteristic display of interpersonal style. This will emerge inevitably in response to the tensions inherent in group life and the individual's characteristic pursuit or avoidance of emotional intimacy, power, and acceptance. (2) Feedback and observations will be generated, illuminating blind spots and potential distortions. (3) These reactions are shared, ideally in a nonattacking fashion. (4) Clarification of distortion follows with the individual obtaining a much more objective picture of himself or herself—how he or she relates and affects others. (5) The individual's opinion of self begins to be more comprehensive and reflects objective, consensually validated reality more accu- rately. (6) The individual exercises responsibility over the presentation of self and assimilates the idea that how he or she relates is in fact a personal choice. (7) Realization of this responsibility induces a feeling of empowerment to change and to initiate new behaviors that are not distorted and that are consensually validated. There is a broadening of the individual's behavioral repertoire. (8) Risk taking and subsequent feedback results in validation of these new interpersonal approaches, leading to change within the group. (9) Change within the group is mirrored by change outside of the group and an adaptive spiral ensues. The process of feedback involves each and every member of the group. This medi- ates against a compliant, passive turn-taking mode in the group. The provider of feedback is invariably much more than just an agent in the therapy of others. He or she is disclosing about self, as well.

Clinical Illustration
Jane, a 29-year-old characterologically difficult woman, was referred to group therapy by her individual therapist who complained that individual therapy appeared to be stagnant. Although a talented artist, the patient was unable to organize herself in any kind of consistent fashion, was frequently depressed, and demonstrated a remarkable capacity to sabotage her own efforts. Her prior therapy had focused on her frustrations in dealing with her world and the way in which "all of her opportunities were wrecked by people around her." She felt that no

one valued her, and she repeatedly experienced criticism with very little support. Jane initially dominated and monopolized the group with her in vivo elaboration of her tendency to overwhelm people through her raw and affect laden expression of intense needs and her description of repeated rejections from her mother and the world at large. She recognized that in fact she was overwhelming at times, but attributed it to her large physical size, a condition impossible to alter, hence likely to cause her considerable ongoing rebuff. She lamented repeatedly that no one ever gave her a chance and that she failed to get the credit due her. For several months Jane intermittently paralyzed the group when she talked. Her response to gentle confrontations that she was monopolizing the group, or that she seemed to be keeping people at a distance through her verbalizations and complaints, led to exclamations that she was only talking because no one else was. It was her way of helping the group move along and once again demonstrated that she was never given any credit for doing "good things." Her tendency to end sessions by suggesting that she was feeling terribly depressed further inhibited the group's willingness to confront her. During this early phase of treatment her continued tenure in the group always seemed fragile. This persisted until, after a long, characteristic exposition, that I., a heretofore timid and avoidant man, responded to Jane that in fact what made her likely to incur rejection was not people's cruelty but, rather, a natural reaction on people's part to her repeated broadcasting of her woes, vulnerabilities, and the crimes committed against her. She made people feel overwhelmed and silenced by her laments about being victimized. Rather than eliciting comfort or compassion, she invited rebuff. He went on to say that he had struggled for a long time deciding whether or not to approach her, scared yet again of a hostile exchange, and then realized that if he did not he would continue to turn himself off to her. Jane dissolved into tears and started for the door in a panic. With much support from comembers and the group leaders she was able to stay. Dan went on to say that he was very glad that she did not leave. He decided that ultimately he would give her his feedback because he was indeed proud of her and could not stand to see her continue to be self-destructive. Furthermore he felt confident that she would in fact be able to hear him out, that she was indeed stronger than she let on, thereby in fact bolstering her much desired need for recognition of some real strength.

This session was clearly pivotal in Jane's treatment. Jane's view of herself as a helpless, mistreated, innocent victim of insensitive and rejecting people was challenged with disconfirmation. She began to recognize her responsibility in inviting rejection by making people repeatedly feel like aggressors victimizing her. What is also noteworthy is that it was pivotal in Dan's treatment as well. The group therapist is able to capitalize on these opportunities by bearing in mind an interpersonal framework for each of the members of the group. In this group clearly Jane was a main player. What was less obvious was that Dan engaged in new, affectively-laden risk taking, and the group went on to evaluate with Dan how it was that he found the courage to confront Jane when others in the group had been frightened. His view of himself as timid, frightened, and needing to always be indirect was also challenged by the affirmation of his boldness.

Activation of the here-and-now requires the therapist to move beyond patiently listening for the emergence of themes and group associations although these serve an important and often illuminating function, in particular during times of group instability. When the group is working effectively, the group process remains a backdrop to the interpersonal transactions within the group. This requires a fundamental shift in attitude on the part of the therapist from a position of abstinence and interpretation to facilitation and feedback. The therapist needs to stimulate this in the members of the group as well. Neophyte therapists often feel inadequate and that in dissonance with their professional image, less capable of actively engaging with the group members in an open and direct fashion. What may feel like manipulation at the outset ultimately is experienced as facilitation when it becomes clear that the therapist's activity is focused on moving the group toward greater and more intimate personal engagement (Dies, 1985). On many occasions neophyte trainees report in supervision, with much embarrassment, that they stepped outside of a position of therapeutic abstinence and responded in a direct, here-and-now fashion to the patients' engagement. Indeed this is exactly what is often required and rather than being a therapeutic error or a sign of unchecked countertransference it is often an essential part of the therapeutic process.

The guidelines for feedback described earlier also relate to the therapist in regard to countertransference. The therapist is both participant and observer. Like others in the group, he or she may get hooked into an interpersonal recapitulation. In fact, Strupp (1980) suggests many therapists fail miserably in containing their hostility in response to provocations by their patients. What is imperative is that the therapist be able to get unhooked, by analyzing his or her emerging emotional reactions, processing them, and putting forward feedback in a fashion that is workable for the patient. It is the therapist's task to find palatable ways of saying unpalatable things in order to help the group move beyond the perimeter of engagement into actual engagement. The therapist will feel more confident with this transparency if he or she is first able to distinguish between reactions that are induced by the patients and reactions that he or she brings to the therapeutic setting. This process is much assisted by the therapist's own personal therapy and self understanding.

Nor should the therapist feel compelled to be transparent with all reactions, recognizing the importance of not overstimulating the group prematurely. It is a means to a therapeutic end and not an end in itself (Dies, 1977). An additional safeguard is the recognition that therapist transparency should serve only the interests of the individual group members' therapy and never the therapist's own personal needs for self-aggrandizement. By the same token the therapist needs to insure that the group does not rely upon the therapist either to initiate feedback or to give the capping conclusion at the end. Each member's feedback is as valuable as the therapist's but the therapist is in the unique position of having an objective view that others may miss. There will be times when the therapist needs to advocate both for the "attacking patient" and for the "attacked patient" (Leszcz, 1989), thereby helping the group identify the subjective experience and distortion that underlies overtly maladaptive behaviors. Confirmation of the effectiveness of the therapist's interventions will be reflected in the group members' increasing personal and affective engagement with one another, increasing group interaction, feeling of cohesion, and capacity of individual members to operate autonomously within the group (Schlachet, 1985).

The concept of bridging (Ormont, 1990) is useful to the therapist as a strategy to enliven the group, decrease disengagement, and increase emotional connection between members. It requires a persistent focus on interpersonal transactions in the here-and-now with pursuit of salient core transactions that are reflective of ongoing patterns within the context of the contemporary relationships. The therapist's objective according to Ormont is to connect one member with another. In a beginning group, a therapist will need to take active responsibility to set this in motion, although a more mature group will be able to do this itself. Strategies include consistently asking questions about observable and inferred engagements and interactions within the group, and verbal, behavioral, and attitudinal resistances to intimacy, with a view to deepening individuals' affective experience within the here-and-now.

Often the greatest challenge to the group therapist is maintaining the group effectively in the here and now. Despite the eagerness for feedback and for hearing from one another how they come across, engaging in the here and now involves a much higher level of exposure and intimacy than is customary in social interaction. Shifting from the content of what is being discussed to the process of what emotions the discussion and the discussants induce in the group members invariably raises anxiety. However, this focus holds each patient's attention to the group, and mitigates against sterile expositions of events that the group knows little about and has little power to effect.

Slife and Lanyon (1991) recommend a shift away from the traditional Western way of thinking of linear causality. To believe that the answers lie in the past invites feelings of victimization and self-absolution. Alternatively the concept of circular causality suggests that the ingredients required to effect personal change are present in one's contemporary life. The idea of "depth" in therapy may need to be reevaluated to promote a shift from the emphasis on genesis to the emphasis on what leads to the broadest and most effective forms of change within the individual. In this process, therapy is demystified. Answers lie not in the past nor in reliance on the therapist, but rather are to be found through a process of responsible, honest, respectful, and collaborative engagement between patient and therapist, and between patient and patient. The therapist in this model of group therapy will be very active but he will be active in the interest of stimulating activity on the part of group members and with the aim of making the group less rather than more leader dependent.

The intensity of the here and now will obviously lead to the emergence of resistances to further engagement and self-disclosure. Frequently this resistance centers on the issue of subjective feelings of safety and vulnerability. Hence a group norm that invites members of the group to move at their own paces and respects differences will be most valuable. It is important to identify in preassessment sessions, issues that are likely to interfere with engagement in the group. For example a tendency toward aggressive bullying as a way of dealing with insecurity, or of compliance and other-serving, if highlighted in the pregroup assessment can often be better accessed subsequently in the group life in the midst of its reenactment. Intervening in order to help the group disengage from yet another repetitive sequence can often be achieved by the therapist inviting group members to step back from their affective involvement. It is appropriate to buy some time until the group members are better able to understand what is going on rather than feel compelled to react in ways that are clearly nonproductive. Intense emotional heat that seems out of proportion with the objective situation is often a very useful signal that some core interpersonal difficulty that reflects on the individual sense of self has been touched. Through its hyper-reactivity, it serves as a marker for central issues. The therapist can ask aloud questions such as the following: What has been triggered? What has been recreated? What has been avoided? What is the benefit to the patient to persist in what is obviously hurtful? Until proven otherwise, each and every comment or question within the group should be viewed as an expression, avoidance, or obstruction to the emergence of the true self of the individual members of the group. Each action or behavior by each member of the group has meaning and the therapist's task is to help all members to pursue this significance. Valuable information invariably follows from the pursuit of the phenomenology of the individual's current experience within the group.

Clinical Illustration

George, a member of substantial duration in an ongoing group, demonstrated recurrent difficulties in maintaining closeness with others. His view of relationships was that allowing himself to become close to someone allotted that person great power over him, power that would be utilized in a sadistic and demeaning way. He had a history of repeated, abrupt job terminations related to aggressive explosions and coworkers' unwillingness to work with him. George relished verbally intimidating people around him. At other times, he complained of feelings of loneliness and isolation. His early course in the group was punctuated by hostile attacks on comembers. One such attack precipitated a comember to say that she was tired of feeling that she was going to be sacrificed in the interests of George's therapy, raising a serious question for the therapist about the group's capacity to tolerate George's aggression. This group was an observed group, and in the early phases of his treatment, observers repeatedly recommended George's termination, an option seriously considered in private by the therapist, who was concerned about the destructive effect of George upon the group. Some of this concern was addressed by the therapist offering a conceptual framework to other members of the group, even at times when George himself seemed unwilling to hear it. His framework focused on George's need to attack in response to his fear that getting close would allow members of the group to attack him. What he wished for was an opportunity for closeness without contamination or hostility, yet by his persistent expectation of hostility and his provocative and hostile testing of the safety of engagement, George made it very hard for people not to retaliate. This retaliation would confirm his worst fear and lead to yet another vicious cycle. In response to feeling vulnerable he made others feel vulnerable. It was suggested that this harmed him in two ways; it invited the actual attack and at the same time made him feel deserving of further attack because of his aggressivity and related guilt.

In a recent stretch of group sessions there was a notable change in George's behavior, culminating in his turning to the group with an overt request for support. The one person he felt close and safe with at work was being transferred. He was sad, soft, and accessible through much of the meeting. He received clear, unambivalent feedback and support for his open disclosure. Later in the meeting he reacted furiously to an objectively benign shift in focus made by Barbara, another member of the group. George perceived Barbara as stealing the group away from him and leaving him bereft in his moment of vulnerability. George persisted in his distortion that Barbara was devaluing and diminishing him, and treating his vulnerability with disrespect. He became progressively more angry and antagonistic and the group experienced a resurgence of the old provocations. In the midst of this sequence of meetings, Barbara's grandfather died, which was not unexpected but still a source of significant grief and loss for her. In consecutive meetings George criticized Barbara for not showing enough emotion and for withholding information from the group about what she felt, at a time when the group was empathizing with her loss and thinking about their own vulnerability to loss. Although there was certainly a kernel of truth in George's feedback, in that Barbara had a morbid shamefulness regarding any display of affect, George's style so polarized the group that this idea was impossible to examine. At one point, in fact, when asked why he looked so distracted while Barbara was speaking, George said that he found her very boring. The group was pushed into an impasse. Barbara tried to finish her work saying that she was not going to allow herself to be derailed by George, an important step forward for her in ownership of her affective experiences, but it was very difficult for people to proceed without addressing George. They turned their attention to him and spoke about their anger at his cruelty, and his unrelenting attack on Barbara at a time of obvious pain for her. George had succeeded in hooking the group and, without intervention, this no doubt would have turned into yet another sequence of George experiencing initial closeness as destructive and dangerous.

The therapist asked the group to try to back away from the heat and to entertain ideas about why George would be so attacking of Barbara. In fact, Barbara protested that she had always been one of the most supportive members of the group toward George, and it felt particularly unfair to her that he would attack her at a moment of grief. Ultimately what emerged through patient feedback to George was that he was doing to Barbara what he perceived she had done to him—when she opened herself up and took a real emotional plunge with the group he pulled the rug out from under her in the same way that he perceived she did to him. Specifically because she had been one of the closer members of the group to him, he experienced that much more anxiety and apprehension that she would attack him in his vulnerability. The therapist suggested that George was convinced that by opening himself up to the group, he would elicit a sadistic attack. He was determined to see the present in terms of the past. His fundamental belief was that the group members would inevitably attack him for drawing closer to them, as he repeatedly experienced his father doing. It appeared that he was finding it impossible to connect the reality of being vulnerable and attached, without the reality of being hurt and attacked, and he was successfully making himself the object of the group's anger in this process. The therapist added that no doubt George could well succeed in completely destroying any sense of connection with members of the group. The challenge to the group was to hold George responsible for his destructive behavior but not to be sadistic—to get unhooked. It was an extremely critical time for the group not to withdraw or attack. George's response to this extensive processing was to say, "I hear what you're saying, but it doesn't seem to penetrate."

The situation was diffused for the time being. In the next session George began by saying that he had been doing a lot of thinking about what had happened in the last several sessions. It was striking to hear how he could experience things so differently from the way everyone else did. Yet the group seemed so clear and persistent, perhaps it was a sign that they were seeing something that he was not. In his associations he added that he recognized within himself a propensity to push people to the limit, in particular people who have been good to him, and he had never been aware of that trend before. This led to his exploring that if he pushed people to the limit, to test his worst fear, he could in fact actualize it. By shifting the group's emphasis to include empathic awareness of his vulnerability, rather than only responding to his overt behavior, the group could begin correcting his distortion that closeness inevitably led to attack. The message was also made clear to George that as the author of his own interpersonal transactions, he could guarantee himself failure if he so chose, and he would have to assume responsibility and appropriate guilt for the destructiveness of his behavior.

This clinical vignette is intended to illustrate the power of the group when it operates in the here-and-now. Illumination of interpersonal behavior, patient distortions, and transferential distortions that individuals make, coupled with the shaping influence they have on their own interpersonal environment, are very evident in George's reactions to the group and his attack on Barbara. A particular strength of group therapy is its provisions of a range of reactions to a common stimulus, thereby deepening the awareness of what each person's subjective contribution is to interpersonal experience. The group's containment and feedback, assisted by the therapist's modulation of the counter-response, interrupts the interpersonal recapitulation. In this instance stimulation of affect was very easy, in fact too easy, and what was required was modulation of the intensity. What was more difficult was the process of cognitive integration and the processing of the events within the group. The sequence of affect evocation, reflected in individuals' characteristic exposition of self and interpersonal schema, coupled with feedback from others, must be followed by a self-reflective loop of processing—the cognitive integration of the experience. This can only be achieved in a group that has reached a level of maturity and cohesion, such that its members can tolerate intense negative affects without group members destroying each other or the group disintegrating. Hence, cohesion is an essential ingredient of the corrective emotional experience. The therapist's own reactions both provide useful feedback to the protagonist and a model for other group members of open, responsible self disclosure, and the rights and limitations that are part of human relatedness.

Conclusion

Interpersonal theory serves as the essential anchor for the interpersonal model of group psychotherapy. By drawing attention to patients' interpersonal worlds, and the centrality of interaction within the group, as both a mechanism for illumination and for repair of interpersonal disturbance, a powerful modality is accessed. In the same fashion that current models of individual psychotherapy emphasize the experiential centrality of the therapeutic relationship, this model of group psychotherapy emphasizes the centrality of peer interactions and consequent, dynamic interpersonal learning.

Looking to the future, it appears the field will be faced with the challenge of providing treatment to a broader range and greater number of individuals, reflecting both societal and economic considerations (Rutan & Stone, 1984). Challenges to be faced by practitioners of this model of group treatment include both outcome research and process research considerations. Are there differences in the nature of improvement produced by different models of group treatment? Does successful outcome at termination of therapy translate into long-term, durable gains? Do the patient's significant others agree that there has been improvement, in addition to the evaluation of the therapist, patient, and research observers? Process measures may include attention to ways in which the core interpersonal patterns can be best illuminated and comprehensively understood within the group. Successful outcome in individual therapy is linked directly to the quality of the therapeutic alliance and the frequency and accuracy of therapist interventions that does confirm the patient's core pathogenic beliefs (Weiss et al., 1986). The parallel elements need to be examined in group psychotherapy. How can the group therapist best facilitate the emergence of group members' central interpersonal patterns and provide disconfirming peer and therapist interactions? What interactions inadvertently disconfirm the individual's core interpersonal schema? The next stage in development may well center on the ability of practitioners and researchers to examine this linkage between process and outcome in specific fashion.

References

Alexander, F., & French, T. (1946). *Psychoanalytic therapy: Principles and applications.* New York: Ronald Press.

Azim, M. F. A., & Joyce, A. S. (1986). The impact of data-based program modifications on the satisfaction of outpatients in group psychotherapy. *Canadian Journal of Psychiatry, 31,* 119–123.

Bellak, L. (1980). On some limitations of dyadic psychotherapy and the role of the group modalities. *International Journal of Group Psychotherapy, 30,* 7–21.

Bion, W. R. (1961). *Experiences in groups.* New York: Basic Books.

Bloch, S., & Crouch, E. (1985). *Therapeutic factors in group psychotherapy.* New York: Oxford Medical Publications.

Dies, R. R. (1977). Group therapist transparency: A critique of theory and research. *International Journal of Group Psychotherapy, 27,* 177–200.

Dies, R. R. (1985). Leadership in short-term group therapy: Manipulation or facilitation. *International Journal of Group Psychotherapy, 35,* 435–455.

Flowers, J. V., & Booraem, C. D. (1990). The frequency and effect on outcome of different types of interpretation in psychodynamic and cognitive-behavioral group psychotherapy. *International Journal of Group Psychotherapy, 40,* 203–214.

Grunebaum, H., & Solomon, L. (1987). Peer relationship, self-esteem and the self. *International Journal of Group Psychotherapy, 37,* 475–513.

Horner, J. A. (1975). A characterological contraindication for group psycho-therapy. *Journal of the American Academy of Psychoanalysis, 3,* 301–305.

Horwitz, I. (1983). Projective identification in dyads and groups. *International Journal of Group Psychotherapy, 33,* 259–281.

Kibel, H. D., & Stein, A. (1981). The group-as-a-whole approach: An appraisal. *International Journal of Group Psychotherapy, 31,* 409–429.

Kiesler, D. J., & Anchin, J. (1982). *Handbook of interpersonal psychotherapy.* Elmsford, NY: Pergamon.

Leszcz, M. (1989). Group psychotherapy of the characterologically difficult patient. *International Journal of Group Psychotherapy, 39,* 311–335.

Leszcz, M., Yalom, I. D., & Norden, M. (1985). Inpatient group psychotherapy: Patients' perspectives. *International Journal of Group Psychotherapy, 35,* 411–433.

Luborsky, L., Crits-Christoph, P., Mintz, J., & Averbach, A. (1988). *Who will benefit from psychotherapy? Predicting therapeutic outcomes.* New York: Basic Books.

Malan, D. H., Balfour, F. H. G., Hood, V. G., & Shooter, A. (1976). Group psychotherapy: A long-term follow-up study. *Archives of General Psychiatry, 33,* 1303–1315.

Merman, G. L., Weissman, M. M., Rounsaville, B. J., & Chevron, E. S. (1984). *Interpersonal psychotherapy of depression.* New York: Basic Books.

Modell, A. M. (1976). The "holding environment" and the therapeutic action of psychoanalysis. *Journal of American Psychoanalytic Association, 24,* 285–307.

Ormont, L. (1988). Resolving resistances to intimacy. *International Journal of Group Psychotherapy, 38,* 29–45.

Ormont, L. (1990). The craft of bridging. *International Journal of Group Psychotherapy, 40,* 3–17.

Rothke, S. (1986). The role of interpersonal feedback in group psychotherapy. *International Journal of Group Psychotherapy, 36,* 225–240.

Rutan, J. S., & Stone, W. N. (1984). *Psychodynamic group psychotherapy.* Lexington, MA: Collannade.

Safran, J. D., & Segal, Z. V. (1990). *Interpersonal process in cognitive therapy.* New York: Basic Books.

Schlachet, P. J. (1985). The clinical validation of therapist interventions in group therapy. *International Journal of Group Psychotherapy, 35,* 225–238.

Slife, B., & Lanyon, J. (1991). Accounting for the power of the here and now. A theoretical revolution. *International Journal of Group Psychotherapy, 35,* 225–238.

Strupp, H. H. (1980). Success and failure in time-limited psychotherapy: A systematic comparison of two cases. *Archives of General Psychiatry, 37,* 595–603.

Strupp, H. H., & Binder, J. L. (1984). *Psychotherapy in a new key: A guide to time-limited dynamic psychotherapy.* New York: Basic Books.

Sullivan, H. S. (1953). *The interpersonal theory of psychiatry.* New York: Norton.

Weiner, M. D. (1974). Genetic versus interpersonal insight. *International Journal of Group Psychotherapy, 24,* 230–237.

Weiss, J., Sampson, M., & Mt. Zion Psychotherapy Research Group. (1986). *The psychoanalytic process: Theory, clinical observations and empirical research.* New York: Guilford Press.

Yalom, I. D. (1985). *The theory and practice of group psychotherapy* (3rd ed.). New York: Basic Books.

Zaslav, M. R. (1988). A model of group therapist development. *International Journal of Group Psychotherapy, 38,* 511–519.

Existential Group Psychotherapy

The Existential Lens

From its inception, the Group Psychotherapy Training Program of the Washington School of Psychiatry has paid attention to what has come to be called "existential group psychotherapy." There is no doubt in my mind that this is due to the influence of one of the founders of the program, the late Hugh Mullen, MD, whose prominence in the field derives from his early applications of existential thought to the problems of psychotherapy. Indeed, in the first Institute (1995), I presented a paper entitled "Some Thoughts on the Existential Lens in Group Psychotherapy," which I dedicated to Dr. Mullen, who had been one of my teachers when I was a student at the school.

By the time of NGPI, Dr. Mullen had assumed faculty emeritus status, but he emerged from retirement to offer brief comments on that paper that April Sunday. Those comments are included in his untitled response, "Notes on April 23, 1995: The Existential Lens." Mullen had published his ideas widely a generation ago; so much of it now is considered mainstream. But we must not be lulled into inattention: Is it *really* so that group therapy can be conducted with one's focus steadily on the irreducible elements of human existence? Mullen had said that these were "birth, intercourse, and death." These papers must make the reader wonder whether it could really be all that simple.

Bernard Frankel, PhD, was once a visiting scholar at a conference dedicated to existential approaches. Though we have not included his papers in this volume due to space, it is worth recalling his approach. He began that weekend with a dispassionate introduction describing the alienation of man, but, as he described his clinical experience for the conference members, his passion became increasingly clear. And what is existential therapy if not passionate?

George Saiger

Some Thoughts on the Existential Lens in Group Psychotherapy*

GEORGE MAX SAIGER

Introduction: The Psychotherapy Relationship

It all began with Sigmund Freud. His conception of psychoanalysis was not existential, but was instead consciously objective and "scientific." Nonetheless, his early focus on the importance of the psychoanalytic relationship was to have an impact on the development of existential psychotherapy. He had first discussed transference as a distortion of the psychoanalytic relationship in the case of Dora (Freud, 1905). He continued to refine his ideas on this matter, delivering them finally as the twenty-seventh and penultimate lecture of his public "Introductory Lectures on Psycho-Analysis" at the University of Vienna in 1916. The Great War was still being fought, and exchange of ideas was seriously limited. Nevertheless, the Lectures were published almost immediately, Part III (which included the lecture on transference) appearing in May 1917 (Freud, 1917). They were widely read, and were quite likely known within the German-reading intellectual community as soon as the war was over, perhaps providing a stimulus for consideration of the ways individuals affect one another. Within a year of the war's end, four major scholars, apparently independent of each other, published on the "dialogic principle," all during 1918–19: Martin Buber, Franz Rosenzweig, Ferdinand Ebner, and Gabriel Marcel. For each, the emphasis was not on intrapsychic distortions of relationships, but on the dyad as an entity in itself, encompassing

---

* This paper was originally delivered, in somewhat different form, at the National Group Psychotherapy Institute of the Washington School of Psychiatry on April 23, 1995. It was dedicated to Hugh Mullen, who had been one of my teachers at the school two decades earlier.

more than the sum of its two parts (Buber, 1918; Rosenzweig, 1976; Ebner, 1980; Marcel, 2002).

Of the four thinkers, it was Buber who caught the attention of the psychotherapy world with his formulation of "I-Thou" relationships (Buber, 1918). This was not accidental. Buber had studied clinical psychiatry in Leipzig as a young man and planned, early in his career, to write a criticism of Freud's work. He never did so, but later he revealed that he had throughout his career maintained a lively interest in the relationship between spirituality and psychotherapy (Schaeder, 1973, pp. 204, 260) It was only after his formal retirement in 1951 that he published for a psychiatric audience, first in a preface (Buber, 1951) to the posthumous publication of Hans Trüb's *Healing Through Meaning* (1951). The next year, the German periodical *Merkur* published an exchange of views between Buber and Carl Jung. In one sense, their debate was about the transcendence of God, but it can also be read as reflecting different views about the nature of human relationships. For Jung, "Thou" was an internal psychological construct and thus modifiable intrapsychically. Buber insisted that "Thou" is radically other, thus creating a relational space not under the control of either party (Jung, 1957; Buber, 1952; Schaeder, 1973).

Jung's own influence on the development of existential therapy was also significant, although in the 1950s this was not yet clear. Years earlier, he too had focused on the nature of relationships in psychotherapy, describing the process as a "dialectic," wherein the analyst and analysand were seen as coparticipants in the endeavor of analysis (Jung, 1935). In using the term *dialectic* to describe the therapeutic relationship, Jung draws our attention to the tension inherent in the cooperative endeavor.

Patients sometimes spontaneously accept this dialectic. The following clinical fragment illustrates one patient's understanding that therapy was not simply a matter of a therapist working on him:

> L.R. is a 38-year-old single male who had left my practice over a year earlier in a fit of paranoid rage induced by medication noncompliance. We had had no contact since. Through other residents of his group home, community nurses, and a case management agency, I had heard that he was back from the state hospital and again living in a halfway house in the community. Through the same channels he knew about my professional activities in the community. Then one day he sent me a postcard in which he addressed me familiarly, although this had not been our custom during the therapy.
>   It said:

> Dear George,

>   Thank you very much for the therapy. It seems you are doing very well. That therapy that we shared must have been something. God Bless You.
>   L.A.R.

In 1957, Buber was a guest lecturer at the Washington School of Psychiatry where he delivered the William Alanson White Memorial Lectures. Leslie Farber, then chairman of the faculty, introduced the published William Alanson White Lectures, focusing on the debt psychiatry owes to Buber's "philosophic anthropology" (Buber, 1957; Farber, 1957). A year earlier, he had delivered a paper titled "Martin Buber and Psychiatry" at the school's Symposium on the Interrelationship Between Religion and Psychiatry (Farber, 1956). In that paper, he linked Buber's ideas to the interpersonalist work of Harry Stack Sullivan. No more an existentialist than Freud, Sullivan, the founder of the interpersonal school of psychoanalysis and of the Washington School of Psychiatry, was concerned about the problem of the overobjective observer. He considered therapists' overzealous attempts to be objective as one of the "parataxic" distortions of the therapeutic relationship. He coined the term "participant observer" to describe the therapist who could alternately engage the patient and then pull back to examine what had gone on (Sullivan, 1953). Farber correctly saw this as an approach to a more mutual I-Thou relationship.

Buber, aware of such connections, chose this school as the venue for the exposition of his broad and clearly nondisciplinary ideas. He had explained to Margaret Rioch the previous year that what was required, for psychotherapy and for other disciplines dealing with human beings, was an absence of dogmatism and a spirit of inquiry. Years later (Rioch, 1986) she remembered particularly how he phrased this idea to her: "When one is 80 years old, one has to choose carefully which places one will go to. There isn't so much time left. I want to come to the Washington School of Psychiatry because it is one of the few places which keeps the questions open."

The lectures, "Distance and Relation," "Elements of the Interhuman," and "Guilt and Guilt Feelings," all work and rework the dialogic principle: the relationship with the other is the key issue of the psyche. The importance of this principle will resurface in this paper as we consider several other streams of existential thought.

Will and the Problem of Meaning

The Denial of Death (Becker, 1974), a critique of psychoanalytic thought, won its author (posthumously) a Pulitzer Prize for general nonfiction the year it appeared. Ernest Becker was not a clinician; he was a cultural anthropologist who taught at Berkeley, San Francisco State, and in Canada about psychoanalysis. In his book, Becker uses the existential lens, as demonstrated by its attention to religious issues, a recurrent focus on the terror of death, and extensive attention to the works of Søren Kierkegaard, the nineteenth century existentialist Danish theologian.

Becker called him "The Psychoanalyst Kierkegaard" to draw attention to the parallels with psychoanalytic concepts. Kierkegaard saw the essential human dilemma as somehow managing to live in the face of the abyss of existential angst. This was accomplished by "faith." "Faith" here encompasses both its current usage of religious belief and also the broader acceptance of culturally defined meanings. For many, faith has a dulling, routinizing effect; for some it fails altogether and the abyss beckons; for the rare "Knight of Faith" meaning can be redefined in heroic ways.

Becker saw Otto Rank as the psychoanalyst who most clearly carried Kierkegaard's work into modern psychology. Rank's incorporation of meaning and will into the practice of psychotherapy is of significant clinical importance (Rank, 1909/1959). Like Kierkegaard, he focused on culturally defined meanings. Unlike the Danish theologian, he eschewed the lofty term "faith," using instead the more startling "lies." A kinder word, which he also used, was "illusions." Neurotics, he noted, had this way of not accepting the civilizing lies, of daring to face the dread of the truth more nearly head-on. The modal case would thus be the characterologically depressed patient who cannot be cheered—and will not be analyzed—out of his/her angst. There is an obvious problem to this formulation: although we all know such people, most real-life patients who form our groups do not conform to this Rankian illusion. More often they are riddled with useless anxieties, or are narcissists who cannot bear giving up power, or are lonely people who fear intimacy. For them too, Rank saw, and Becker applauds, the utility of helping them face the necessities of their lives—necessity subsuming both the possibilities and the limitations. Rankian therapy embodied a kind of pre-AA serenity prayer: the goal, in the usual translation from Rank's German, is "the voluntary affirmation of the obligatory." Rank's biographer, Jim Lieberman, has pointed out that the real power of the idea comes through better with rendering the German in simpler language: "willing 'yes' to the must" (Lieberman, 1985).

Jung, it should be noted, would have disagreed. In his Answer to Job (1954), he argued that it was up to man to change the meaning of his/her life, not to fulfill it. For a time, I adopted a stance based on this idea. I suggested to patients who were nervous about entering group therapy that they were starting with a fresh slate; that they could introduce themselves as they liked to the group, even changing their names if they wished. I promised not to blow the whistle on them. Not one took me up on the offer. The reason, as the patients well knew (and I should have), is that there are certain "musts" to an individual's being within which s/he must live, even in the psychotherapy group.

Becker ultimately concluded that mental health means to stop lying. In so doing, he unfortunately slipped away from the tragic starkness of Rank's insight. As we try to endow existence with meaning, we make approximations, assert our illusions, that is, in the Rankian sense, we lie. The goal of psychotherapy is to reformulate the lies, that is, reformulate the attributed meanings that make raw experience comprehensible, in ways less likely to cripple. The reformulation is a process; old formulations, reinforced by accrued defenses, are given up only grudgingly. When this occurs in psychotherapy, and especially in a psycho-therapy group, defenses must be accorded considerable respect. Of course they can obstruct human fulfillment and prevent engagement with a therapy group. The art is to learn to what extent defenses have an adaptive value. Ann Landers repeatedly advises unhappy wives: "Ask yourself whether you'd be better off with him or without him." Rankians would ask the same about ego defenses. The task of the existential therapist is not only to work within the dialogic relationship, but also to do so with an understanding of the interplay between the must and the defense that can facilitate the least restrictive solution.

There is no small measure of irony in seeing both Rankian and interpersonalist psychotherapies as part of the existential approach. When Rank's practice became "Rankian," he stopped considering himself a psychoanalyst. In 1930, he was stripped of his honorary membership in the American Psychoanalytic Association. The motion to do so was introduced by A. A. Brill, a classic Freudian (no big surprise!). What should give us some pause is that it was Harry Stack Sullivan, the pioneering interpersonalist, who seconded the motion (Lieberman, 1985).

Object Relations and Existential Psychotherapy

We have come this far without offering a definition of "existential psychotherapy." It indeed eludes definition, leading us to rely on metaphors such as "faith," "lies," and "philosophic anthropology" to convey its meaning. A working definition offered by Goldenson in The Encyclopedia of Human Behavior (1970) is as good as any:

> Existentialism focuses on the inner core of man, as opposed to the emphasis on outer adjustment . . . the essential problem of existence is that of . . . being oneself.

The attention of object relations theorists to very early experience, occurring prior to any verbal or conceptual organization of the world, makes their work important to the existential therapist. For example, Winnicott's (1953) focus on the transitional experience, which develops out of the first infantile projections and identifications, is conceptually close to this undifferentiated core. Eigen (1993) has asserted that both the transitional experience and Winnicott's later concept of object usage (1963) represent "areas of faith." "Faith" as Eigen uses it, reflects experience that is undertaken with one's whole being.

Bion (1963, 1967/1994, 1970), as group therapists know, began elsewhere, but in time he arrived at the Kierkegaardian abyss, and looked at it through the eyes of the infant. The raw, inchoate, sensory impressions that bombard the organism, Bion called β elements. There had to be an α process by which these were transmuted into α elements, that is, mental impressions. Thus psychic life begins. Myths, dreams, language, concepts, all organize these impressions. The organization of any given individual psyche is at once enabling and restrictive. It enables one to live in the physical universe, but a variety of neurotic and not-so-neurotic experiences limit the correspondence between the psychic representational scheme and the world outside. Within the paranoid-schizoid position, reorganization is difficult, if not impossible. The restrictions are modifiable, however, whenever the depressive position is attained.

Bion had the idea that knowledge was of two fundamentally different sorts. He coded them as "K" and "O." K knowledge is cognitive: examples would include knowing one's multiplication tables, knowing one's lover's tastes, knowing the developmental history of one's patient. Beyond that was the ultimate 0. 0 is not something known; it is something experienced. At times, 0 is understood by what it is not—it is not a piece of mastery, it is not a parental introject. It seems apparent that Bion means this as a sort of religious truth; his language often parallels religious language when he tries to describe it.

To the extent that 0 is conceived of as an "ultimate reality" to be discovered, Bion seems more essentialist than existentialist. I think that this would be a misreading, however. Bion did not conceive of 0 as "out there" waiting to be discovered. He made the critical observation that 0 evolves as the subject tries to get at it—truly an existential dialectic. An important task of psychotherapy would be to identify false approaches to the ultimate reality of 0.

Bion also uses the notion of 0, oddly enough, to express a practical, K knowledge-related principle: 0 is the emotional truth of a therapy session. How peculiar! The one facet is Kierkegaardian darkness and formlessness. The other, useful side, central to the enterprise of group therapy supervision, is "the group theme!" In a way, I tease Bion's shade here, because all this mixing of therapeutic technique with Ultimate Meaning verges on blasphemy. But Bion is never to be dismissed lightly. It may be precisely here that he helps us. Group therapists, after all, must have an appreciation of the group's life, the ground upon which the multiple and fleeting figures of group interaction become manifest. 0 is appreciated differently by different therapists, depending on individual style and temperament. For some of us, this is intense, experiential, and preverbal. For others it is more helpful to allow an admixture of some degree of K knowledge so that the experience can be understood.

Logotherapy

"Logotherapy," the therapy of meaning, derives from Viktor Frankl's experiences in a Nazi death camp where he existed for several years during World War II. Indeed *Man's Search for Meaning* (1984) was written in 9 days in 1945 and initially titled "From Death Camp to Existentialism." It has since been translated into 20 languages; my 1984 edition was the 73rd English-language printing. Despite Dr. Frank's moving and fervent statement of the importance of meaning attached to the future, I was caught by allusions in the book to an earlier pre-Holocaust version of his thought. Frankl had brought a manuscript with him to Auschwitz, managing to smuggle it past two checkpoints before he lost it at the delousing station. "This is my life's work," he explained to an ultimately unsympathetic trusty during those hours. A play of emotions was revealed on the veteran's face: confusion, pity, amusement, mockery. Then he bellowed, "Shit!"

At that moment, Frankl wrote, he understood that his whole prior life was erased. As it turned out, though, it wasn't totally so. He managed to keep a sense of meaning during the years of brutish concentration camp life that followed. One way was by preparing himself psychologically for the reunion with his wife (even though part of him knew that she had already been done away with by the Nazis). Later, he worked to reconstruct the manuscript, writing notes to himself on scraps of paper that were liberated with him in 1945. He saw that there came a time for many inmates of the camps when any sense of purpose in living would disappear. They would give up, lie in their own excrement, indulge some deferred pleasure, like smoking an illegally obtained cigarette, and die. Frankl came to understand that survival required holding on to a belief in the meaning of the present as it touched future goals.

"I call it logotherapy," wrote Frankl, because "logos is a Greek word which denotes 'meaning.'" Well, yes, but λογος more commonly means "word," as in John I: "In the beginning was the Word and the Word was with God and the Word was God . . . and the Word became flesh and dwelt among us, full of grace and truth, and we have beheld His glory, glory as of the only Son from the Father."

Rank had taught us, remember, that words are lies. The point was echoed by Frankl's contemporary, Kenneth Burke (1961), who coined the term "logology," the study of words, around the same time that Frankl published his "logotherapy." Burke's thoughtful book demonstrates how language functions to organize perception and experience. When Bion's 0, itself ineffable, becomes attached to a word, λογος, comprehensible meanings can adhere to it. Frankl appreciated this, as is evident from the three facets he identified in the concept "existential": existence itself (i.e., the specifically human mode of being), the meaning of existence, and the striving to find a concrete meaning in personal existence, that is to say, the will to meaning.

The second facet addresses the problem of meaning that has been the focus of the preceding pages. The third facet addresses Frankl's approach to therapy. He drew a parallel between his "will to meaning" and the presumed "will to pleasure" in Freudian thought and "will to power" in Adlerian psychology. Freud would have objected that the linking of the concept of "will" with the pleasure principle was a tendentious artifice. I believe he would have been right; the centrality of will is not Freudian, but Rankian. Frankl locates its expression in creation, in love, and in suffering. It can be frustrated, leading to what Frankl calls an existential vacuum and thus to psychopathology. We will return to the application of this idea to group psychotherapy below.

The Existential Group Psychotherapist

Hugh Mullen, MD, was among the pioneers of modern group psychotherapy. He was denied certification by the American Institute for Psychoanalysis in 1953 because all his analytic patients had been, by his own design, "contaminated by group." He turned this to his advantage 3 years later when he became the seventh president of the AGPA. During his tenure, the AGPA Institute was created, forming the genesis for the small experiential study group.

Studying what went on in groups led Mullen to increasing discomfort with the continual efforts to describe group process by invoking ever more creative reworking of Freudian concepts. The creative approach he developed seemed to him to flow from the tradition of existential philosophy, and he came to see himself as an "existential group psychotherapist." Because of his influence, we, his students, were taught that Morris Parloff's (1969) classic tripartite classification of group therapies into "intrapersonalist" (now more commonly called "intrapsychic"), "transactionalist" ("interpersonalist"), and "integralist" ("group-as-a-whole") needed to be expanded by one: "existentialist." That belief has endured at the Washington School into Dr. Mullen's semiretirement.

In 1964, he and Iris Sangiuliano published *The Therapist's Contribution to the Treatment Process* in which they described the essence of their belief about what was different about group therapy (Mullen & Sangiuliano, 1964). The key was a different breed of therapist. In individual psychotherapy, the therapist might well cultivate dependence and/or a transference neurosis for therapeutic ends. But in group therapy, Mullen believed, the therapist had to abandon such status ploys and role plays. S/he needed to strive to be honestly there with his/her patients. For Mullen and Sangiuliano, Heidegger's concept of dasein (i.e., being there) was central. It was what made them existentialists. Such dasein subsumed several components which they presented as "modifications of traditional concept, theory, method and goals" to the Conference on Existential Psychiatry at the American Ontoanalytic Association in New York in 1960: the establishment of a more certain bilaterality between patient and therapist, the continuous activation of change in the therapist, the enhancement of immediate experience, the expression and use of the therapist's subjectivity, the identification in therapy of the "ethic of integrity, the availability for psychotherapy of the many groupings of patient(s), and therapist(s), e.g., patient groups, family groups, married couple groups, and multiple therapy (two or more therapists).

We, his students, had a dilemma. Hugh Mullen was not one to be there with us in our sophomoric skepticism about his ideas, be it based on allegiance to traditional analytic training or, more likely in those days, based on our infatuation with the "group-as-a-whole" outlook which then dominated the department. Mullen lectured from a prepared text and then entertained questions (which had better not be too confrontational). This did not seem to us at all like Sartre or Camus. Indeed, Mullen never meant it to be: he remained unimpressed with "existential therapies" and didn't much like Yalom's book on existential psychotherapy (Yalom, 1980) when it came out. He argued that the crux of the matter was that the therapist, not the therapy, be existentially there.

Much of what was a radical redefinition of the therapists' contribution to the treatment process in 1960 is now considered standard practice across a broad spectrum of dynamic practice. Such is the price of success. Indeed, newer psychotherapies that abrogate patient-therapist bilaterality in the service of stimulating a planned transference reaction or, in cognitive therapy groups, of teaching new modes of cognition seem boldly revolutionary. Not only has bilaterality come to be widely accepted as a principle, so have the use of subjectivity, the sensitivity of the therapist to countertransferential interferences and the willingness to work through them (i.e., to change), the value of the here-and-now, and the openness to trying out different frames. All are now commonplace.

Much less accepted is the explicit emphasis on integrity and ethics. No one puts out a shingle advertising nonethical therapy, but ethics, like any other aspect of the work, can be compromised by inattention. In today's climate, such inattention has become more common and thus more serious. Control of patients for some greater good has come to seem quite reasonable, both in and out of forensic psychiatry, both in and out of managed care. Over the years, Mullen's thought has moved toward more explicit examination of this component. In a recent paper (1991) he considered the problem of "Inherent Moral Practice in Group Psychotherapy." By that time, having applied himself to the formal study of philosophy, he saw morality in psychotherapy as emerging from the principles of existentialism. He distinguished between "benevolence," the love of the other, and the practice of "beneficence," a well-doing to others, which he called "exactly the exercise of patients in group psychotherapy." Mullen pointed out that patients seem to take to mutual self-help easily, perhaps instinctively. This is also my experience; during the preparation phase for entering a psychotherapy group, prospective patients foresee it as an exercise in helping others. This perception is a decidedly negative one for many, especially those who see themselves as suppressing their own needs in order to help others. For good or for ill, the perception is there, both for the therapist and for the patients, suggesting that such morality is inherent in the group. Mullen argues that it is incumbent upon the therapist to match the group's morality with both benevolence and beneficence. Being there isn't good enough; the therapist has to honestly find a way to like being there.

Early on, Mullen identified professionalism as an important component of therapist morality. He noted that "some believe," and no doubt he is among them, "true professionalism is only achieved when the therapist denies him- or herself, in order to care for others" (Mullen, 1991, p. 195). The example he cites is attendance at workshops and seminars and personal group psychotherapy, all performed at some sacrifice. He would no doubt agree to include the careful reading of this article as another example of such laudable behavior.

Ultimate Concerns: The Fear of Death

Irvin Yalom was already a decade past the first publication of Theory and Practice of Group Psychotherapy (Yalom, 1970) when he published Existential Psychotherapy (Yalom, 1980). He did not reference Mullen's work, but did acknowledge his debt to similar ideas in the humanistic psychology of others (Rollo May, Carl Rogers, and Abraham Maslow) who had also wrestled with healing the cleavage between doctor and patient. He defined existential psychotherapy by its content rather than by the therapist's stance: "Existential psychotherapy is a dynamic approach to therapy which focuses on concerns that are rooted in the

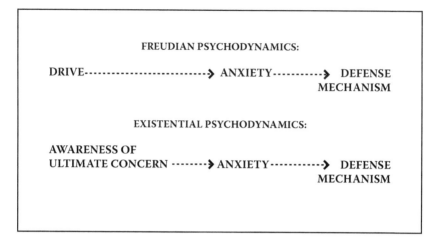

Figure 1   Existential psychodynamics (Yalom).

individual's existence" (emphasis his). He considered it "dynamic," and therefore in the mainstream of psychodynamic therapies, because, in his conception of it, it dealt with forces in conflict, as his schematic adaptation of the Freudian model shows (see Figure 1).

Yalom asserted that the four ultimate concerns to be worked with were: death, freedom, isolation, and meaninglessness. There is of course nothing sacred about this list; it comes after all from a contemplative kind of knowing, perhaps enhanced by pondering the great philosophies of dead White males. Mullen had proposed a similar, but triune, division: birth, intercourse, and death. Freud's two ultimate instincts, eros and thanatos (i.e., death of the individual and procreation of the species), could also be read in this context. Charles Schulz runs an ongoing thread in the comic strip, Peanuts, playing on the perspective of his somewhat self-absorbed character, Snoopy (see Figure 2).

The point is not to pick the winner of the "ultimate concerns game," but rather to underscore that Yalom developed a not unreasonable list that he then discussed in clinical terms. I commend to you his discussions of all four ultimates, but for

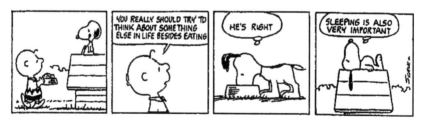

Figure 2   Snoopy's ultimate concerns (PEANUTS reproduced courtesy of United Cartoonists, Inc.).

purposes of this paper, I'd like to focus on one, the fear of death, to illustrate how we might work with this lens.

Psychological attention to the fear of death was not new. It had already received special attention by those who worked with populations where death loomed large. In one of the earliest contributions to the then hardly existent field of geriatric psychotherapy, Balint (1951) had chosen a particularly eloquent label, *Torschlusspanik* ("the panic at the closing of the gate"), to describe this phenomenon in the elderly. For Balint and other students of the psychology of aging, this panic represented a manifestation of late-stage narcissism, and as such, an obstacle to psychotherapy.

Existential therapists, Yalom among them, understood that awareness of the fear of death was not an obstacle. Instead it represented a therapeutic opportunity. In the fifth chapter of his book, Yalom presents a 9-page clinical vignette describing the introduction of a patient who had an untreatable cancer with a 3-year prognosis into an ongoing general therapy group of six other, apparently healthy, adult outpatients. This was not accidental. Yalom the therapist was by this time very interested in how the issue of death would play out in a group that he, an interpersonalist at heart, thought of as a social microcosm.

The microcosm he described was comprised of seven patients typical of those seen often in everyday clinical practice. He described five briefly. Several were caught in transference situations the resolution of which was due to the encounter with the dying man: Lena, who had been orphaned preoedipally, reexperienced her childhood longing for a protector and rescuer; Don, who was locked into an ongoing power-based transference struggle with Yalom; and Ron, who had wavered obsessionally for much too long over the issue of termination. Two other patients, recognizing in the dying man the fleeting of time, became able to express love to significant others in their lives.

Yalom described the sixth patient, Sylvia, in more detail. She was obese, insomniac, alcoholic, asthmatic, and depressed. At first, she was angry with the cancer patient for not trying hard enough for a cure for his illness. Her anger became more easily touched off in general; then she suffered a panic attack, then a chemical sensitivity, and then a relapse from sobriety. She became conscious of the suicidal quality of much of her behavior. After some months of such strategies, she tried to encounter the cancerous co-patient more directly. Anxiety rose sharply and ideas of quitting the group became strong. Yalom came to see her as struggling primarily with "death anxiety" and its attendant defensive maneuvers. With this, she became aware of much death-related ideation and of memories of death. A desperate, dependent, demanding, and ultimately frustrating transference was resolved. She was no longer overcome by fears of annihilation and could successfully terminate.

And the cancer patient himself thanked the group for saving his life. He didn't mean that he outlived the grim prognosis, which he did; but that they helped him restore an honest affectivity. His survival at first had depended on its suppression as he submitted to the necessary diagnostic tests and treatments, but this had long since become counterproductive.

The clinical vignette illustrates several steps toward this good outcome: Yalom was first of all interested in the problem. He attended to death-related themes as they emerged in dreams, in the there-and-then accounts of the group members, and what is most important, in the here-and-now activities of the members. Within the life of the group, there was a developmental sequence of working with the anxiety that a dying member introduced. First there was avoidance. Then came a period of defensive grappling with the fears around death, manifested by displacements, denial, distortions, projections, etc. Once the defenses could be minimized, death anxiety could be experienced and its existential reality accepted. A richer experience of life could then be experienced within the group. It seemed then to follow, without much work on anybody's part, that gains were applied to relationships on the outside.

Yalom considered these and many individual cases where fear of death/longing for death/denying death are the central issues. Being an "ultimate" concern, it is ubiquitous. A question then forces itself upon us. How, if it is so central, do we miss it so often? Yalom devoted three short paragraphs to the central issue of therapist denial. Even when dealing with groups of the dying, or the already dead, as in cancer support groups, AIDS groups, or groups of Holocaust survivors, therapists experience markedly little anxiety about death themselves. In the name of supporting the healthy defenses of the patients, we can too easily justify our own avoidance of death anxiety, thereby keeping things safe. This happens repeatedly in therapy groups and in experiential training groups. The references to death that come up do not become the focus, if a safer issue can be substituted.

I managed to colead an AIDS group for 2 years without losing any sleep, as the guys talked endlessly about the side effects of antivirals, the discrimination gay men face in accessing care, and costs of the newest herbs from Africa. Yalom would suggest that my good cheer should have been a signal that propelled me back into personal therapy or into supervision in order to confront my resistance. I suspect he would be the first to agree that the short shrift he gives countertransference issues in his book reflects that he shares with me—and here I consciously echo Becker's commanding title—the denial of death.

Frankl's style in group therapy was very different from Yalom's. In *Man's Search for Meaning* (Frankl, 1984), he treats us to a clinical vignette of a therapy group as part of his discussion on how he works with the will to meaning in psychotherapy. A patient was admitted to his service who had two children: one was severely crippled from polio; the other, her golden child, died. I too have such a patient, an elderly gentleman suffering from post-CVA depression whose physician son had died unexpectedly several years before. His only remaining heir is a chronic schizophrenic son, a continuing burden instead of a source of support for the aged father in his hour of lonely chronic suffering. My patient rails at the numerous injustices of nursing home life and wishes to die; Frankl's attempted suicide. In the therapy group described by Frankl, the woman tells her story. Frankl, the therapist, then turns to another group member and asks her to imagine herself at 80 years of age, childless but socially prominent and wealthy. The patient complies. He turns back to the index patient, who can now see that each life has a mission; hers is the care of the polio-afflicted son. Then he addresses the group-as-a-whole and asks the members to imagine whether apes in a scientific lab appreciate the meaning of their suffering. The group replies "of course not." The therapist then links this to human suffering and asks the group, "Is it not conceivable that there is still another dimension, a world beyond man's world; a world in which the question of an ultimate meaning of human suffering would find an answer?"

This vignette stirs mixed reactions. This clinical maneuver is an example of refraining or cognitive restructuring. For it to succeed as a therapeutic intervention, there must be a strong idealizing transference at work. That may well have been the case. How could his patients, how could we, withhold admiration, even idealization, from a Holocaust survivor, one who developed this method from his own experience in Hell? Still, experience attests to the variability of transference manifestations in groups. However gratifying it is to one's narcissism to believe that the transference is one of idealization, there are always other possibilities. It seems quite possible to me that many of the quick cures that Frankl describes, including this group vignette, are based on the unwillingness of the suffering patient to challenge the illustrious doctor with doubts or reservations. Easier by far to thank him for his cure, swallow the disappointment, and continue to muddle on, confirmed in one's isolation.

That conclusion is even clearer in another case Frankl presents, this time from his individual therapy practice, wherein he quickly cures a depressed Orthodox rabbi whose children have died. The therapeutic technique was an earnest presentation to the patient, a trained Torah scholar, of maxims from folk religion around the issues of death and afterlife. Cross-cultural psychiatry has taught us that this kind of insensitivity cannot work, The only viable conclusion left to us is that the idealization of the therapist, in that case at least, existed, but not in the mind of the patient after all.

To resolve the dilemma we must integrate the existential therapist with the existential therapy. The transference trap can be avoided in these situations if the therapist attends adequately to his subjectivity, as Hugh Mullen argued. If one can enter into being with the bereaved suicidal patient, and only if one can enter into being with the bereaved patient honestly and courageously, then, and only then, can there be some credibility to a joint search for some meaning beyond the pain.

As to my own bereaved patient, I had expected a dramatic existential therapy. Instead, I found myself being with him through long periods of complaints about nursing home management, how bad the food was, side effects of medications, and the frustrations of physical therapy. We dealt with minor issues of empowerment, such as trying to go out occasionally for a restaurant meal. There was hardly a word about the dead son from either of us. Surely I did not try to instruct him in the meaning of his tragedy. In the second year of treatment, I was able to encourage him to attempt a trip to visit his grandson. We talked about the trip for two or three sessions. Just as I was to leave for the nursing home for our last visit before his scheduled departure, I received the news of the sudden death of a young adult son of close friends. My feelings were a jumble then; I was not in a state that could be called "self-aware." I knew I was frightened and confused. I debated whether to tell my patient of my distress. There would have been some advantages to this course: it seemed likely that I might be perceptibly distracted; I was also well aware of the personal meaning it would have for him. Since my motivations for self-disclosure seemed fuzzy at best, I decided against revealing. Instead I asked how he was doing. He responded, after a few pleasantries, with "Did I ever tell you my boy was adopted?" This was followed by the tearful recounting of anecdotes from his son's childhood and early adulthood, about support the young man had given him during earlier family crises, and about his final illness. He ended by asserting his intention to shower the grandson with gifts during this trip and to visit the son's grave—alone. I never did say out loud why I thought I could be with him on that day. Nor did I share the speculation with which I end this paper: that my ability to be there, unusual and unspoken, allowed a major step in working through.

Conclusions

There turns out to be no single lens that provides a way of viewing existential psychotherapy. In this paper we have considered four vertices: (1) the importance of relationship in therapy; (2) the focus on meaning; (3) the focus on very basic human experience; and (4) existential therapy as that therapy in which an existentially aware therapist works. Though conceptually distinct, these viewpoints overlap in clinical practice.

Much of contemporary dynamic psychotherapy has absorbed these ideas. This isn't surprising, given their roots in the earlier analytic theoreticians. This is especially true of the first vertex, the centrality of relationship in therapy. The interpersonal approach to group therapy, which encompasses far more than existential therapy, is grounded in this context (Leszcz, 1992). To a lesser extent this is also true of the fourth vertex, which we have here identified with the work of Hugh Mullen. That does not reduce Mullen's ideas of bilaterality to merely historical interest, however. In today's market, an emphasis on definable goals in psychotherapy, with severe limitation of time and topic, has reemphasized what the therapist does to the patient.

Within the excitingly diverse field that is group psychotherapy today, one would expect existential work to be done by those therapists who consider themselves interpersonalists. Among these, there are some who are especially tuned to issues of meaning and/or ultimate human experience, however defined. They are today's existential group psychotherapists.

Professor Buber, we are still trying to keep the questions open.

This paper was originally delivered, in somewhat different form, at the National Group Psychotherapy Institute of the Washington School of Psychiatry on April 23, 1995. It was dedicated to Hugh Mullen, who had been one of my teachers at the school two decades earlier.

References

Balint, M. (1951). The psychological problems of growing old. In *Problems in human pleasure and behavior* (pp. 69–85). London: Hogarth.

Becker, B. (1974). *The denial of death.* New York: The Free Press.

Bion, W. (1963). *Elements of psycho-analysis.* London: Heinemann.

Bion, W. (1970). *Attention and interpretation.* London: Tavistock.

Bion, W. (1994). *Second thoughts.* Northvale, NJ: Jason Aronson. (Original work published 1967)

Buber, M. (1918). *I and thou (Ich und Du).* New York: C. Scribner.

Buber, M. (1951). Introduction. In H. Trüb (Ed.), *Heilung aus der Begegnung.* Stuttgart: Klett.

Buber, M. (1952). Reply to C. G. Jung. In *Eclipse of God.* New York: Harper.

Buber, M. (1957). The William Alanson White memorial lectures (4th series). *Psychiatry, 20,* 97–129.

Burke, K. (1961). *The rhetoric of religion: Studies in logology.* Boston: Beacon Press.

Ebner, F. (1980). *Das wort und die geistigen realitaten (The word and spiritual realities).* Frankfort: Suhrkamp. (Original work published 1919)

Eigen, M. (1993). *The electrified tightrope.* Northvale, NJ: Jason Aronson.

Farber, L. H. (1956). Martin Buber and psychiatry. *Psychiatry, 19,* 109–120.

Farber, L. H. (1957). Introduction to The William Alanson White memorial lectures (4th series) by Martin Buber. *Psychiatry, 20,* 95–96.

Frankl, V. (1984). *Man's search for meaning.* New York: Simon and Schuster.

Freud, S. (1905). Fragment of an analysis of a case of hysteria. *Standard Edition, 7,* 3–124. (Original work published 1901)

Freud, S. (1917). Introductory lectures #XXVII. *Standard Edition, 16,* 448–464.

Goldenson, R. N. (1970). *The encyclopedia of human behavior: Psychology, psychiatry and mental health.* Garden City, NY: Doubleday.

Jung, C. (1935). Principles of practical psychotherapy. *Collected Works, 16,* 3–20.

Jung, C. (1957). *Reply to Buber.* Spring. Zurich: Spring Publications.

Jung, C. (1960). *Answer to Job.* New York: Meridian Books. (Original work published 1954)

Leszcz, M. (1992). The interpersonal approach to group psychotherapy. *International Journal of Group Psychotherapy, 42*(1), 37–62.

Lieberman, E. J. (1985). *Acts of will: The life and work of Otto Rank.* New York: The Free Press.

Marcel, G. (2002) *The philosophy of existentialism.* Citadel Press. (Published posthumously)

Mullen, H. (1991). Inherent moral practice in group psychotherapy. *International Journal of Group Psychotherapy, 41*(2), 185–197.

Mullen, H., & Sangiuliano, I. (1964). *The therapist's contribution to the treatment process: His person, transactions and treatment methods.* Springfield, IL: Charles C. Thomas.

Parloff, M. (1969). Analytic group psychotherapy. In J. Marmor (Ed.), *Modern psycho-analysis* (pp. 492–531). New York: Basic Books.

Rank, O. (1959). In P. Freund (Ed.), *The myth of the birth of the hero and other writings.* New York: Vintage. (Original work published 1909)

Rioch, M. J. (1986). Fifty years at the Washington School of Psychiatry. *Psychiatry, 48,* 33–44.

Rosenzweig, F. (1976). *Per Stem der Erlosung (Star of redemption).* Haag: Martinus Nijhoff. (Original work published 1918)

Schaeder, G. (1973). *The Hebrew humanism of Martin Buber.* Detroit: Wayne State University Press.

Sullivan, H. S. (1953). In H. S. Perry & M. L. Gavell (Eds.), *The interpersonal theory of psychiatry.* New York: Norton.

Trüb, H. (Ed.), (1951), *Healing through meaning.* Stuttgart: Klett.

Winnicott, D. W. (1953). Transitional objects and transitional phenomena. *International Journal of Psycho-Analysis, 34,* 89–97.

Winnicott, D. W. (1963). The development of the capacity for concern. *Bulletin of the Menninger Clinic, 27,* 167–176.

Yalom, I. D. (1970). *The theory and practice of group psychotherapy.* New York: Basic Books.

Yalom, I. D. (1980). *Existential psychotherapy.* New York: Basic Books.

Notes on April 23, 1995
The Existential Lens

HUGH MULLEN

I like the term *lens* for describing the various kids of group therapies. This denotes differences in treatments and differences perceived by the patient, by the therapist, and by the objective observer. If one is an existential therapist, and insofar as one is an existential therapist, the following characteristics to some degree might be present.

The therapy that you offer your patient must be a different experience for them, one that he or she cannot find anywhere else.

Your own personality—you yourself—must be used or employed in your treatment time.

An existential treatment can only be offered insofar as you yourself are existential—or to the degree you are existential. It cannot be just another method applied. In a sense it is not so much a method but more a way of being with the group. The groups that frequently focus on birth, death, intercourse, and commitment are many times existential in nature.

Existential treatment centers on the patient's existence and its meaning to him. The following concepts instruct the therapist:

- The patient is free.
- The patient's destiny, his therapeutic change, is within his own power.
- The patient's only hope is in acting (thinking, feeling, and doing.)
- The patient is his own future.

Under these conditions of freedom and responsibility, the patient's life is not only possible but also meaningful.

Psychoanalytic Approaches

Psychoanalysis in Groups

In a sense all our work is "psychoanalytic" in that it rests on the psychodynamic thinking with roots in Freudian analysis. But as the papers in this volume amply demonstrate, the emphasis in most of the approaches we teach has developed into very different theories and methodologies, some of which have a decidedly *non*-psychoanalytic cast. We have thus found it valuable to reaffirm the insights that ground us. Leon Lurie, MS, the most senior member of our faculty, has chaired conferences at the Institute with a psychoanalytic focus. His paper "Theories Are Ideas" applies to all the theoretical ideas included here, but Lurie sees his work as essentially psychoanalytic; woven into his short paper are many classical psychoanalytic ideas such as therapist abstinence, countertransference, and regression.

The "psychoanalytic" conference of the Institute takes on a much different flavor when it is chaired by Stewart Aledort, MD, who has developed what he calls "therapist-centered therapy."

In his paper, "A Model for the Development of an Analytic Culture in Intensive Multiweekly Group Psychoanalysis" and in his demonstrations at the Institute, he shows a thoughtful yet exciting application of this approach to group work. A second, briefer, paper by Dr. Aledort is included in the section on systems approaches, in which he discusses the similarities of his approach with that of Yvonne Agazarian's "systems-centered therapy."

The first time that Anne Alonso, PhD, visited our Institute, she had only recently published her dramatic paper, "The Shattered Mirror: Treatment of a Group of Narcissistic Patients." She spoke several times that weekend, once on "The Shattered Mirror Revisited," once on "On the Analytic Action in Group Therapy," and once on "The Dream in Analytic Group Therapy." Any one of those could have rightly found its place in this volume. I have chosen the last in part because of its unique focus, in part because of the carefully crafted terse explication that illuminates both the theoretical and the practical problems of working with dreams in analytic group therapy.

George Saiger

Theories Are Ideas

Leon Lurie

Theories: contemplation or speculation, guess or conjecture.

—*Random House Unabridged Dictionary*

Tiger got to hunt,
Man got to sit and wonder,
"Why, why, why?"
Tiger got to sleep,
Bird got to land;
Man got to tell himself he understand.

—Kurt Vonnegut, *Cat's Cradle*, 1968, p. 124

In 1988 Anton Chekhov wrote "The Lady With the Dog," a short story that ended with "You can't figure out anything in this world." A fellow writer objected: He wrote Chekhov: "That finale is abrupt; it is certainly the writer's job to figure out what goes on in the heart of his hero; otherwise his psychology will remain unclear." Chekhov responded: "I take the liberty of disagreeing with you. A psychologist should not pretend to understand what he does not understand. Moreover a psychologist should not convey the impression that he understands what no one else understands. We shall not play the charlatan, and we will declare frankly that nothing is clear in this world. Only fools and charlatans know and understand everything."

A professional paper includes references to previous workers in the field of interest. This gives a scientific aura to the authors' ideas that helps all concerned to entertain the notion that we are dealing with something like facts. We seem to need this illusion—as if we can hardly bear to know how little of the mysteries of personhood can be apprehended. So we make up stories about and to our patients and each other. We call these stories theories in order to soothe our troubled, ignorant spirits. And then we reify these theories to further bury the unknown— the unknown that we find unbearable.

But this creation and reification of the calming theory becomes a straightjacket. The original soothing function turns to dullness. It stultifies our wide-eyed, open-spirited curiosity about the miracles around us. Our lively gaze is deadened.

Almost any professional paper will reveal this tendency to talk about ideas as if they were facts of life. More than that, our entire profession is based on the notion that help for the patient lies in finding underlying meaning and understanding of the conscious and unconscious motives, feelings, et cetera, of the troubled person. We have surmised that this finding of underlying meaning is curative. This idea (fact?) goes back at least as far as Freud. Perhaps it would be best not to tamper with it. Maybe our powerful human need for meaning in life will not be denied. But I can't help wondering if it would not be enriching for us and our patients to be more tentative in our approach.

But aside from the problem of willfully pretending to ourselves that ideas are facts, we find another problem. If we assume that ideas are facts we are assuming a posture that puts the therapist in the position of the knower. It encourages all parties to view the helper as omniscient and omnipotent. The therapist's one-up position is reinforced. Is this good for the patient? If the therapist is one-up, how does this affect intersubjectivity? It is easy to be confused about the nature of our therapeutic intersubjectivity if we are not clear about the implications of the one-up position.

The therapist together with all of her feelings and attitudes is as much a part of the field of inquiry as is the patient. If the one-up position is a fact that the therapist is only vaguely, or not even vaguely, aware of, then the therapy involves an unconscious element that must get in the way of the work. But suppose she is aware of her superior position. She can be more complacent about it or less complacent about it. Both these possibilities also present problems.

In the first instance, she assumes the medical model—the doctor is—and, she feels, rightfully—in a superior position. She knows better than the patient what is needed. Moreover, that idea gives her the authority to get the patient to follow orders.

The second possibility—that the therapist is not so complacent—presents us with other complexities. Therapists, like everybody else, cherish and need all the power they can have over people, including their patients. (It may even be that some of us entered the profession, partly or, gasp, even primarily for this reason.) They may, if they are particularly insecure, need to emphasize their power over the patient, not realizing that they can hardly give it up. And if they could, the patient wouldn't let them.

All of this brings to mind the basic question that has been asked forever. What in analytic therapy are the helpful elements? If you believe, as I do, that the relationship is a core element, then maybe the one-up position needs work to see if its dimensions can be reduced or its manifestations can be softened. At the very least we can be aware of the fact and alert to its effects on the therapeutic process.

For example, a new patient found my usual work methods disagreeable. He wanted to express his feelings repetitively on the subject of his seemingly hopeless quest for sexual recognition from his female chiropractor. My comments were empathic, but I also talked about things that were going on between us, such as the fact that he never looked at me when he spoke. He found these interventions irritating, and wished I would shut up. I thought I would for a while. He appreciated my acquiescence, and then, after a bit, got bored with the hours in which he held forth almost without interruption. I think he needed to assert his authority, (he later told me that he had contemplated quitting with me) and it led us to a beginning relationship in which, after a few hours, he asked for more time.

Getting back to theories are just ideas, I do not mean to derogate the need for theories. We could not do the work without some organizing principles. The material coming at us from our patients would be too confusing for us to bear. We need something to help us with our anxiety—not knowing what is happening in the room. We need ideas (which we call theories) to help us make some kind of tentative sense out of the data that we receive from our patients. But the operative word is *tentative*.

To be tentative in doing psychoanalytic therapy means to cultivate our own abstinence. We have to keep our therapeutic ambitions from showing, whether we are in a dyad or a group. The other day a patient came in saying, "I'm all fucked up. I made an appointment with a client for 4:30, the same time as my hour with you. I remembered just in time to cancel it." Now one need not be a brain surgeon to know that forgetting an appointment with the analyst is probably significant, but, controlling myself, I kept quiet, (abstinence) and kept my face in repose. We spoke of different things and the session went along. Finally, about 15 or 20 minutes before the end of the hour the patient said she plans to quit therapy in 4 weeks. She then told me that she spoke to a friend of hers (who happens to be a colleague of mine), who said that forgetting her appointment was not just a lapse of memory, which my patient knew herself, but of which she needed to be reminded. She (or was it they?) thought it meant that she should quit with me. We had enough time to talk about this and she decided not to quit. Like so many of us, my patient wants to be a cherished and well cared for tiny thing, at the same time that she wants to be a self-sufficient adult who can take perfectly good care of herself. This requires from the therapist a delicate balance of full empathic attention combined with a fine-tuned appreciation of what your patient is capable of doing (sometimes with a little stretching) on her own.

Doing group therapy requires, I think, an even more rigorous abstinence on the part of the therapist. Here you have, if the group is on task, many therapists. In my experience, their influence on each other is more productive of new insights than most of what the therapist thinks and says. Last week, to my chagrin, I ignored my own precepts about tentativeness and abstinence. I got an idea in my head about what the group members were doing or rather not doing. This idea came to me after an individual hour with one of the members, and when the group met, I barged right in with my idea. The ensuing silence was deafening. Adding to my folly, I then went on to cite my evidence, which was not inconsiderable. More silence. I finally caught on when somebody said that Leon seems different today, and somebody else, after more silence, started on another subject. By now, a third of our time had gone. I kept quiet and the members did their work for the rest of the session, during which I entered into the discussion with an occasional comment.

Perhaps this vignette leaves you with the same question that it did me: What in the world was going on with Leon that made him act in this unlikely fashion? Possible answers to this question are the stuff of supervision, which makes supervision a close kin to psychoanalysis. We are dealing with unconscious motivation. This material can be worked by oneself, with a colleague, or with a supervisor. But the main point in a case like this, and in most cases, is to realize that something was not right in the first place.

What has this story to do with theory being ideas? I think quite a bit. I used my theory that (1) the group and individual therapy are seamless and (2) that the group creates a valence for actions in individual therapy. Also I was entranced by my multiple evidence that my theory was borne out by the individual work with different group members. These theoretical considerations reinforced an unconscious need that pushed me to barge in, which need I am only now getting a handle on. My unconscious agenda required me to forget that theories are ideas, and ideas need to be borne out by the emerging data rather than vice versa.

To summarize: The conversion of ideas into theories that are then reified into facts is a manifestation of the all-too-human need to know that which is unknowable—what Leslie Farber called willfulness (willing the unwillable). Unless we curb this almost overwhelmingly powerful desire, we get in trouble doing psychoanalytic psychotherapy. We follow our theories instead of following our patients: "You can't figure out anything in this world" (Farber, 2000).

The patient is not responsible for the formation or existence of the group but after his entrance he is very soon responsible for "the fact it (the group) is what it is." His challenge is to change it. In a similar fashion to the Kantian "Categorical Imperative," he must begin to "act on maxims which can, at the same time, have for their object themselves as universal laws of nature."

Reference

Farber, L. H. (2000). *The ways of the will: Selected essays.* New York: Basic Books.

A Model for the Development of an Analytic Culture in Intensive Multiweekly Group Psychoanalysis

Stewart L. Aledort

All group therapists strive to have their groups become what Bion (1961) has described as the "Work group." In the model of group psychoanalysis that I will describe here, the analytic culture of Foulkes (1975) is equivalent. I believe that it is crucial to develop and maintain the analytic group culture if the deepest work of analysis is to occur. The model I propose, which is based on the developmental model of Mahler, Pine, and Bergman (1975), is used in intensive, open-ended group therapy conducted by either a solo therapist or cotherapists two or three times weekly. In group therapy based on this model, the analytic culture can both develop and nurture itself continually.

The analytic work consists of the resolution of preoedipal and oedipal conflicts, mediated through the interactions between the group members, the group as a whole, and the leaders. The narcissistic injuries that underlie many of the personality disorders and the early negative parental introjects are worked through, and new internalized structures are put into place. In my experience, most patients can achieve a complete analysis in group therapy patterned after this mode.

Many group therapists have written of the possibility of doing psychoanalysis in a group format. Wolf and Schwartz (1962) conducted group psychoanalysis but did not use the full impact of the group as an analytic tool. Foulkes and his followers have used the group to activate the analytic process. Roberts and Pines (1992) in their recent review of the group matrix elaborate the therapist's task but do not specify a formal unfolding of the group process. In this paper, I will demonstrate the necessary phases that the group, the leaders, and the individual members must negotiate in order to develop an analytic culture.

Underlying this approach is the assumption of omnipresent, early developmental failures, epitomized by patients containing and holding onto pathological split-off parts of their parents and roles in the family group. These patients have served as family heroes, caretakers, protectors, or scapegoats. All have been, in fantasy, and still are omnipotent children. The preverbal, introjected, pathological conflicts seem to exist independently of cognitive growth and reality testing. They are fed by narcissistic investments and have become part of the archaic grandiose self (Kohut, 1971).

Group Model: The Beginning

The process begins in the first consultation. After the determination of symptoms and syndromes affecting the patient, and the addressing of any immediate medication requirements, an evaluation is made as to whether a patient will require long-term therapy for resolution of the underlying problems and is likely to benefit from group therapy. If so, the modality of group psychotherapy is offered and explained. This educational process has a dual focus: (1) to discuss the individual's conflicts, object relationships, and areas of vulnerability, which will emerge in the group, and (2) to discuss the group setting, which allows members' life "scripts" to emerge in an atmosphere enabling empathy, nurturing, and growth. Such scripts reflect patterns of intrapsychic and interpersonal functioning that served protective functions in childhood but are pathological and ineffective in adulthood. Generally, the entering patient hopes that therapy will enable his or her script to become more efficient and workable, rather than changing it.

The group contract is explained and includes: a minimal 1-year commitment to twice-weekly or three-times-weekly sessions with no alternative forms of therapy and no individual contacts with therapists for any reason. Individuals are allowed a fixed number of free sessions each year. Confidentially is the rule, and extra-group socialization among group members (which is seen as acting out) is forbidden. The rationale for this group contract has evolved over many years of therapy.

Prior to group entry patients are evaluated by the cotherapist (cotherapists are always female social workers), and a concurrence is reached about appropriateness for group therapy and a specific group. Often the cotherapist does the initial interview.

In order for the analysis to proceed, all outside distractions must be minimized as much as possible and all the work must be done within the group boundaries. Although splitting between therapists can cloud therapeutic issues, cotherapy splits within the closed space of the group enhance members' learning opportunities. The group never meets without at least one therapist present, and even though the therapists' interactions within the group are real, we never purposefully reveal our personal lives. All of the above help to create an atmosphere in which the group members can express themselves freely and spontaneously.

Group Composition

These groups are optimally composed of eight members balanced by gender. An attempt is made to include borderlines and narcissistic character disorders in each group and to exclude no patients unless they are actively psychotic. New start-up groups can begin with as few as five members, but we quickly try to reach eight members.

Phases of Group Psychoanalysis

Four distinct phases are necessary for the effective development and functioning of the analytic culture. They can be described as phases of developmental growth (with accompanying regressions) which affect the patients, the therapists, and the group as a whole.

The phases are as follows:

- The FIT
- SEPARATION-INDIVIDUATION
- SEXUALITY, AMBIGUITY, AND SAFE HARBORS
- ANALYTIC CULTURE

Phase 1: The Fit

The TASK/GOAL of the first group phase is to develop a fit and mutual adaptation between therapists and individual patients similar to the adaptation and fit that develops between mother and child, which is the central task of infancy. Such a fit between mother and child requires a mutual adaptation of bodies, inner sensorium experiences, potentials, and capacities (Greenspan & Greenspan, 1985). In the opening phase of the group, the therapists are the sole focus of the new group members. Other group members are obstacles in the way of cathecting the therapist/mother of infancy. Group members attempt to adhere to and get inside the mothering figure; the therapists must accept this penetration and what is inside the group. This process has been referred to as containment (Foulkes, 1975) and is crucial in allowing the development and flow of all the other phases.

The first phase establishes the conditions that enable the central tasks of analysis to take place. The only important connection during the first phase is the meeting of the eyes and bodies in a healthy feeding environment. The outside world does not really exist until a good-enough fit is perceived as possible in fantasy or is established within the group boundaries.

Therapists' Behavior   Through their comments and silences the therapists force the group to acknowledge their need to look at only one of them. One therapist is selected and this therapist becomes the representation of the symbiotic mother. The selected therapist must be able to contain all that is present in the group. During this phase the cotherapist acts as a supportive parent to both the group and the symbiotic-mother therapist, making comforting statements about the difficulty of the task and reminding the group of the frustrations and painful affects that the process requires. The symbiotic-mother therapist constantly reminds the group that he/she is the most important person in the room and will actively intervene when the group tries to avoid him/her and join with other patients. At times he/she will say that the group would rather play with each other in order to deny that they would rather play with him/her. The symbiotic-mother therapist, at least once or twice per session actively reminds the patients of his/her presence and their yearnings toward discovering who he/she is and wanting to know what is inside of this mother. This technique fosters regression, demands aggression, and encourages the idealized parental imagoes to flourish. It also allows a strong group cohesion to develop around the need to be close and inside in a mutually loving and exploring symbiosis with the mother therapist.

In this phase, the therapist who is the symbiotic mother is indulging him and herself in their own narcissistic fantasies; the therapist must be constantly aware of the danger of loving him or herself too much and forgetting that he/she is the recipient of transference feelings, not real feelings. He/she could easily avoid the aggression in the group or become omnipotently silent and act like a guru. The silent therapist at this time could be perceived as depressed or empty as one who must be filled and rescued by the group members.

Group Behavior   In this phase the group is quite tenuous and most of the time feels as if it will not survive. The group typically acts like an infant that isn't being fed enough or changed often enough, or, is held too tightly or not tightly enough. The members are afraid of falling, starving, and lying in their own mess. They chafe under the rules, hate to pay in an orderly fashion, don't like the chairs, complain about the temperature of the room, and don't want to come on time. Their affect is either irritable, whining, or frustrated, and only occasionally are they contentedly smiling.

Content/Issues of Group Sessions   The major issue in this phase is the group's need to find the right fit with the therapists, not with each other, and to acknowledge their lifelong inability to find good fits with their own bodies. As the group experiences the therapist as holding and exploring their irritabilities, longings, and injuries, it feels comforted and wants to work harder and move on. The form and structure of this task are the questions that permeate the group on all levels. Whose group is this anyway? Why are we here, does the room fit right, and are the rules and boundaries to be taken seriously? These questions are made verbal by the therapists in order to frame the task of the group. The group begins to develop a group identity around shared awestruck feelings and mutual distrust toward the idealized parental imago of the symbiotic mother. She can easily alternate between the good mother and the witch mother. Group cohesion begins to form, based on the mutual toleration of aggression within the boundaries of the absence of projected pathological conflicts from the therapists.

Duration of Phase and Transition of Next Phase   The initial phase can last from 8 months to a year. All the phases seem to take longer in groups that meet twice instead of three times a week. Apparently the regression and aggression can be contained and held more comfortably in the more frequent group. The transition to the next phase occurs when the "group envelope" (Day, 1964) appears. The patients are now more possessive about group identity and process. They tend to notice who is present and want the door closed, and a group recorder and historian emerge—all signs that they are moving into the second phase.

Phase 2: Separation-Individuation
The TASK/GOAL of the second phase is the group's establishment and declaration of its own independence; simultaneously, the therapists allow this transfer of power to occur in an orderly and appropriate manner. The archaic grandiose self of the group and the therapists must be replaced by mutual mirroring. With the good-enough mothers in place in reality or fantasy, the group will expect encouragement for autonomous strivings but will also expect resistance from the therapists. The task for the group is the exploration of magical thinking of early childhood, which expresses surprise and wonderment at both the separation from the symbiotic mother and the discovery of their own genitals. The group must learn now to look at each other with intense curiosity and excitement but without action and panic, and to shift from looking at the symbiotic mother in wonderment and awe and fear.

Therapists' Behavior   The therapists must now actively encourage and interpret the group's outpourings in the frame of the group's striving for autonomy and ownership. If such comments are not made, the group will grind to a halt and stay regressed in the earlier phase; it will keep repeating earlier dramas until the therapists recognize the need to advance or the group dies. The therapists must encourage play and not see it as a resistance to hard work; instead, they must see it as the work of the group. The therapists must reconnect with the child in them: they must be able to play and become excited and childlike without losing the mature cognitive skills that the group relies on at all times. They must be the objects of magical fantasies and yet contain the excitement in the group's bodies.

The therapists' task is also to surrender their omnipotent narcissistic position of Phase 1. This difficult task is rife with danger. They must suffer loss and emptiness without retaliating or expecting the group to fill them up and thus help them to recapture the earlier idealization and grandiosity. A therapist could easily be sadistic, punishing the group for abandoning him and playing amongst themselves. The cotherapists are now more vulnerable to acting out with each other in order to deny the narcissistic losses. They may project rage onto each other, or they may fall in love with each other, which could even lead to their separation, fusion, or departure from the group.

Group Behavior   During this phase the group is basically asexual and dyadic in its object relations. The members are not as irritable and infantile and now feel more like apprehensive little children, wanting to know if it is all right to be excited by their discoveries, both in their bodies and in their thoughts. They can easily be injured if they are denied their rights and yet still feel very beholden to the therapists for permission. An example follows:

A patient in a group in the early part of Phase 2 angrily moved a vase of flowers that was obscuring his line of vision to another patient. In the past he had been provocative, demanding that his grandiosity be admired and becoming terribly injured when it wasn't. His moving the therapist's vase was seen as another grandiose act by the group. His rejoinder was to state clearly that he could move the vase since this was "our group" and his needs were realistic. The therapists acknowledged that he was right, pointing out that his and the group's anger expressed the group's ambivalence about claiming the group as its own.

During this stage the group also is intrigued with its discoveries and suffused with magical thinking. Here is an example:

On a coffee table in my office stood a hollowed-out papier-mâché duck and a cluster of small cut-glass animal figurines. Over time, the duck was filled with a floral arrangement and a small glass mouse was moved to another part of the room. One female member who had been basically silent for the first year, awakened to the discovery that the duck must have eaten the mouse. She knew it was a fantasy, yet it held important meaning for her and the rest of the group. Other groups that met in the same room didn't notice the change at all. This group, led by the patient's fantasies, was entranced and kept returning to her ideas. There were dreams of men with chicken-like breasts, of Thumbelina dancing on little fingers, and of men leaping tall buildings. Thumbelina eventually became the little girl's clitoris, and much later the duck that ate the mouse was replaced by the mother who swallowed the enthusiasm and early excitement of the little girl. She later dreamt that she had given birth to a bag of ice (her own perception of her stony silence in the group), but a live fetus followed, which was her new emerging warmth and excitement.

Content/Issues of Group Sessions   The basic content of the group during this phase consists of anxieties and excitement over attempting something new either outside or inside the group. The patients begin to bring in their dreams, which seem to symbolize the discoveries themselves. Considerable embarrassment, giggling, storytelling, and joking occurs, and the group members begin to ask personal questions of each other and look to each other more frequently. There is also an omnipresent threat of regression to the symbiotic mother, and the group makes various attempts both to ward her off and yet keep her alive. This ambivalence is particularly manifest around the time of action. The emergence of the group recorder and historian serves to give the group its own identity, yet they also remind the group of its infantile behaviors and many times the members act out the symbiotic mother when the therapists refuse to play the role.

The hidden grandiosity in the group is in the patients who won't separate because they are there to rescue the therapists from their narcissistic losses. The tensions around separation issues create anxiety as both the excited explorers and the clingers to mother demand of each other undying love and admiration for their staked-out, narcissistically invested positions. As a result, sibling arguments occur frequently and are interpreted now as reflections of the previous narcissistic positions. There are memories both of great moments in their lives and of great failure and shameful events. Masturbation themes become more evident, along with shame and embarrassment. Prideful feelings are fragmentary and tenuous at best.

Introduction of New Member   New members find entering the group during this phase particularly difficult. The new members are a threat to the newly dis-covered and fragile autonomous self and stir up the group's longings to return to the symbiotic phase. As the therapist interprets the material in this vein, the group allows the opening phase for the new members to continue. Empathy for the new members' plight becomes an important ego function for the group. At times scapegoating occurs with a new member or even with an older member. The scapegoating—which is an inevitable reflection of earlier unconscious expe-riences—allows the group to hold on to the gains artificially while projecting the negative, destructive affects into the other. These negative projections are cherished, experienced as an act of great love and intimacy, and are fueled by the narcissistic investments of their omnipotent and pathological self-idealization.

Duration of Phase and Transition of Next Phase   This phase can last at least 1 year because there is constant regression back to the earlier phases plus the accep-tance of the new patient's right to have his or her own first phase. The transaction is not as dramatic as the envelope formation, but it is heralded by the awareness of the sexual differences between the members and the concomitant discovery of the father in the room through associations and through the clear awareness of the cotherapy team as male and female.

Phase 3: Sexuality, Ambiguity, and Safe Harbors
The TASK/GOAL of the third phase is the group's introjection of a safe harbor from the regressive pulls toward the symbiotic mother and from the fantasized retaliatory preoedipal mother, who experiences the group as disloyal to her. The group must allow the father to come in as the protective parent in order for this process to ensue. The group must also deal with the discovery of the sexual differ-ences between the members and the concomitant anxieties, fantasies and ambi-guities. The early aspects of object-drive sexual fantasies and bodily experiences are reenacted and reexplored. The observing ego and the capacity to laugh at one's own reenactments begin to flourish.

Therapists' Behavior   The therapist's role during this phase is to help facilitate dreams, fantasies and object attachments while at the same time ensuring a safe harbor from the enraged, abandoned, preoedipal parent. Both therapists now must question aggressively the group's need to keep them in the role of the retaliatory parent and help the group members recognize their denial of anxiety over the discovery of the other sex and their fantasies toward each other. The therapists actively encourage any movement of the members toward each other and their mutual fantasies of interest. The therapists' vulnerabilities lie in their need to stay in the center as the abandoned angry mother and in their resistance to the group's urge to couple and be sexual. Like the group, the therapists must allow the father to enter and must allow themselves to be coupled off. This may lead to conflicts within the therapy couple and acting out. Because the group now has many more active fantasies about the therapists' lives, their interactions with each other, and how they work, the therapists may want to stay in the earlier phase of play and denial of their sexual feelings toward the group members. These sexual feelings must be dealt with in the context of the group's sexual emergence in order for the sexual therapists to appear in a form that protects them and enables them to function as the group's safe harbor. The therapists' ability to acknowledge and laugh at their own mistakes and peculiarities is an important ego function for the group now, providing a model for the development of the group's sense of humor and excitement.

Group Behavior   The group is suffused with the excitement and anxiety of noticing the sexual differences between themselves and the therapists. They are searching out objects to cathect the libidinal and aggressive drives as well as a place to project what was introjected into them. The depressed, abandoned parent makes herself known through the self-selected patient who demands to be dealt with. This patient contains and holds the preoedipal depressed and angry parent that the group members need to dispel from inside themselves. His sacrifice must be acknowledged to protect him from himself. The group's need to stay loyal to the depressed, abandoned parent is seen in their polarization of the sexes and denial of the sexual differences, and the suffocation of excitement.

In one of the groups, two women banded together and proclaimed themselves sisters who would gladly kill all the men and were quite adamant in their sisterhood for many months. They shared dreams of togetherness where one would do the killing and the other would defend her in court. There was great homoerotic excitement in these fantasies, and both were in reality asexual at that time in their lives. The homosexual attachment to the angry, depressed, retaliatory parents was denied in consciousness. Eventually the sisters came apart when one would no longer adhere to the oath of homosexuality, which was cloaked to look like aggressive and murderous asexuality.

Content/Issues of Group Sessions   The basic content of the group during this phase is the search for a safe place in which they can cathect each other and project into each other what they introjected. There is much discussion of their fathers, previously seldom mentioned. The intense ambivalence toward the fathers is striking as they acknowledge their longings for him. Memories of early discoveries of sexual differences fill the room, and they recall their early fantasies of where babies come from. The distortions of these fantasies and memories are flushed out, and links to the present distortions in their sexual images of themselves and others are affirmed. Much corrective work is done, which helps advance the members toward further object ties within the group with much less anxiety. Concerns about homosexuality are prevalent, and the group's longings for affection and holding from the same-sex parent cause a great deal of apprehension. The father's appearance offers a chance for a safe harbor, but for the men it is also an awakening of dangerous homosexual longings. These longings parallel the group's need to notice its narcissistic investments in the ambiguity and denial of genital differences. The working through of uncertainty about the insides of the genitals is an important developmental task that the group must accomplish before moving on (Kestenberg, 1968; Bak, 1968).

The narcissistic issues in this phase are the grandiose fantasies of having and owning the only genital in the world. The notion of women as castrated men, the fantasy of phallic women, the anxiety over penis and womb envy, all tend to be fueled by narcissistic investments and are not given up easily. They tend to mask the homosexual longings and dependent yearnings that are held contemptible.

Anxiety and regressive pulls run high in this phase because the patients painfully begin to realize that they are stuck with what they have. They can't go home again and can only attach with their pathological introjects. They must leave the safe harbor of aggressive asexuality and denial of sexual differences. Some members leave at this time, resulting in a profound sense of loss in the group. The lost members reflect the longing and ability to return to the symbiotic mother and highlight the failures and emptiness in all of them.

As the observing ego becomes more dominating and attachments safer, the sheltering harbor is introjected and the revengeful parent becomes less real. The real danger now resides in their own need to treasure their introjects and pathology.

Introduction of New Members   New members entering during this phase are the subject of contempt that is a projection of the group's distaste for their homosexual and heterosexual longings. They also can become scapegoats for the group's anger at its need to stay connected to the depressed, abandoned parent. On the other hand, they also can symbolize the newfound excitement of discovery and be welcomed effusively. A new member can become the long-sought libidinal object that was not present in the group prior to his or her arrival. As a result the new member can feel that he is quite important in the group's functioning and may not want to deal with his own issues and his own phases. He needs to be rescued and reminded gently of his own problems. The group's need to cathect to objects may frighten the new member, and the therapists must be sensitive to these anxieties. The new members may also feel that the group is too close, too familiar, and too sexy for his depression and self-involvement. The group again has to make room for him and develop empathy for his status.

Duration of Phase and Transition to Next Phase   This phase, too, can last for a year. The regressive pulls, the search for the safe harbor, and the working through of the early fantasies of sexual discovery make this a very productive and exciting phase. The next phase is heralded by the group's realization that the danger in their lives lies in their need to treasure the pathology and invest it narcissistically. This and the development of the observing ego and humor and excitement all push the group to the final phase—the analytic culture.

Phase 4: Analytic Culture
The TASK/GOAL of the fourth and final phase of development is the working through of the characterological, instinctual, and object-related conflicts within the patients. The prevalent narcissistic conflicts and their attendant compensatory restitutions are worked through as well. The archaic grandiose self shifts to a more mature self-representation, which then allows for more mature, satisfying object relations. Empathy for others and for the other gender becomes more palpable, and empathy for the little child in themselves surfaces. Homosexual anxiety is reduced, and the patients can often tolerate more envy of their successes than before treatment. Their capacity to hold on to a depressive position (Kernberg, 1974) allows real grief work to occur. Their final task is to terminate from the group in an orderly, appropriate manner, which allows time for grief, admiration, envy, and pleasure to be absorbed and experienced. The ultimate task is to allow the analytic culture to continue while old members leave and new members enter.

Therapists' Behavior   The therapists' role is once again to encourage the development of full-blown complex, transference couplings, using themselves as objects of attachment and reenactment. The therapists many times are the objects of last resort when other group members refuse to join someone in the reenactment. These transference demands can be quite intense, and cotherapists can be of great help to each other in sorting out their roles in the dramas.

In one of my groups, my cotherapist repeatedly warned me to set limits on an angry borderline patient who was terrorizing the group and me. I was going to cure her single-handedly and was reveling in my countertransference rescue fantasies. When the patient threatened to throw an ashtray at me, I was forced to surrender my reverie and begin to analyze with her and the group what had been reenacted, including my role in the drama.

The narcissistic issues for the therapists in this phase are their potential reluctance to take part in the dramas that the group and the patients demand of them. The therapists may not be comfortable being the seductive mother, the sadistic father, the depressed parent, or the revengeful sibling. When the therapists refuse to occupy a role, the group can become gridlocked and angry. The therapists must be able to communicate their roles in the drama and suffer the possible humiliation that is entailed.

The therapists must be comfortable letting members leave and take pleasure in seeing parts of themselves in their patients. They must also be able to tolerate grief at losing favored members and the anxiety that the group will never be the same again.

Group Behavior   The main themes are the group's conscious, eager desire to work and to resolve the conflicts that brought them to therapy. They demand that all the members be present so that the dramas can proceed. They talk about when they are going to leave and remark that this is the best family they ever had. Their ability to understand their own roles in the drama of their lives increases exponentially, and their developing sense of cooperation manifests itself as they allow complementary transferences to emerge. Humor is used to soften the blows of the losses and disillusionments, without resorting to contempt, compensatory omnipotence, and grandiosity.

This is when one notices major changes occurring in the patients' lives outside and inside the group. The results of the hard work come to fruition. Members change jobs, get promotions, start new careers, get married and divorced, and invariably change friendships. Gender ambiguities are resolved, and they generally feel like new persons inside.

Content/Issues of Group Sessions   Couples and triangles dominate the group's atmosphere, and talk of love, hate, revenge, envy, lust, murder, and sex becomes the language of the group. New relationships are formed, old alliances are shattered, and new respect for each other's hard work and difficult histories is manifested. Emergent symbolic events, phrases, dreams, and fantasies capture the group's attention and become organizing foci for the work of resolution. The therapists must pick and choose which of the many dramas fighting for space in the group will take precedence while at the same time referring back to the other latent dramas.

Ambivalent feelings toward individual member's terminations cloud the room all the time during this phase. The transitions are intense and necessary for the life of the group. Fantasies of a group newsletter and of all members leaving at once repeatedly crop up. The sadness, sorrow, and pleasure in the terminations intensify ego growth, which in turn pushes the group to move on. The patients who are ready to terminate usually become surrogate therapists, who at first are scorned and then ultimately admired for their accomplishments. They have to deal with the narcissistic injury of knowing they will be replaced. In the end they struggle to accept the ideas that they weren't loved as they wished, weren't able to rescue as they hoped, and weren't able to maintain the omnipotent child in themselves and in the therapists.

For example, a patient who had been chronically depressed finally found a woman to love, but he loved her ambivalently and tenuously. She left him, and he had to struggle then to realize that he couldn't have it both ways: "He can't both love his depression and her at the same time." In another example, a woman who was involved with a difficult man complained endlessly about his rigidity. She was relieved when the therapists showed her that he had to put up with her phobic conditions as well as that she was "no picnic to live with."

The profound complexities of the inner life are discussed and recognized with great relief; for some patients such realizations arrive for the first time without shame and humiliation. The superego becomes less harsh or more appropriately present in the group as well as in the patients. The aggressive and libidinal drives are split off and brought under better control as relationships in the group change. The patient's previous ability to take all projections without discrimination changes as they work out the pathological projections and introjects in the group. There is a real sense of fullness and freedom when the patients can finally reveal theft inner fantasies, daydreams, wishes, and excitement.

Introduction of New Members   The fate of new members who enter in Phase 4 is even more complex than that of new members who entered during Phases 2 and 3. How do these patients negotiate the developmental tasks that the others accomplished when the group was embryonic, so long ago? One answer is that inherent in all our therapy sessions are hints of all phases. Initially, as I pointed out for earlier phases, the expression of empathy and support for the new members becomes an important ego function for the group. The therapists can also use interpretations that are symbolic characteristics of Phase 1: that is, longing for the good mother, and the dread of the witch mother, to clarify for the new patient what he or she is feeling. At the same time we ask the group to deal with related affects on a more oedipal level. Interventions of this kind can provide a bonding bridge (Ormont 1992) between the new patient and the group.

As the new member becomes more comfortable in revealing problems, she or he may form a mutual attachment with an older member. The therapists' adroit fostering of such coupling can, for example, bolster the new patient's tentative revelations and helpfully channel the stirred up regressive rage in an older patient.

By the use of such protective and integrating measures, the therapists can thus help the new patient to become a full-fledged member of the mature group, remembering early traumata and working to understand its influence on current functioning.

Conclusion

This paper has presented the necessary steps and theoretical underpinnings for the establishment and maintenance of the analytic culture in a particular model of multiweekly group psychoanalysis. The four phases that were described coincide with the phases of psychosexual development and with the narcissistic development line. This model can act as a barometer for therapists, letting them know where they are and what should be happening in the midst of a complex group process. Each phase has its own tasks and structure that can aid the therapist in his search for a way through the maze group process.

The analytic culture takes approximately 3 to 4 years to develop, but once developed can help in the exploration of all the developmental phases for old and new members alike. This model also reaffirms the group as an effective treatment modality for severe-to-moderate characterological patients as well as neurotic disorders. I hope that the model can take some of the mystery out of the therapist's roles and tasks in the group process.

References

Bak, R. (1968). The phallic women: The ubiquitous fantasy in perversions. *Psychoanalytic Study of the Child, 29*, 191–214.

Bion, W. R. (1961). *Experience in groups*. London: Tavistock Publications.

Day, M. (1964). The group envelope. Paper presented at the American Group Psychotherapy Association.

Foulkes, S. H. (1975). *Group-analytic psychotherapy*. London: Gordon & Breach. (Reprinted 1986, London: Karnac Books)

Greenspan, S., & Greenspan, M. (1985). *First feelings. Milestones in the emotional development of your baby and child. From birth to age 4*. New York: Viking Press.

Kernberg, O. F. (1974). Mature love: Prerequisites and characteristics. *Journal of the American Psychoanalytic Association, 22*, 743–769.

Kestenberg, J. S. (1968). Outside and inside, male and female. *American Psychoanalytic Association, 16*, 457–520.

Kohut, H. (1971). *The analysis of the self*. New York: International Universities Press.

Mahler, M. S., Pine, F., & Bergman, A. (1975). *The psychological birth of the human infant*. New York: Basic Books.

Ormont, L. R. (1992). *The group therapy experience*. New York: St. Martin's Press.

Roberts, J., & Pines, M. (1992). Group-analytic psychotherapy. *International Journal of Group Psychotherapy, 42*, 469–494.

Wolf, A., & Schwartz, E. K. (1962). *Psychoanalysis in groups*. New York: Grune & Stratton.

The Dream in Analytic Group Therapy

ANNE ALONSO

We speak of sleep that knits the unraveled sleeve of care. But at the same time Shakespeare was all too aware of how frightening the dreams of troubled people can be, as he puts into Hamlet's soliloquy, "To sleep, perchance to dream, ah, there's the rub"; Hamlet later says, "Oh God, I could be bounded in a nutshell and count myself a King of infinite space, were it not that I have bad dreams" (1 lm ii, 259).

Is there a concept more intriguing than dreams in analytic thought? Beginning with Freud's confidence that dreams are the royal road to the unconscious, we have sought to find deeper meanings for our work with our patients in the dreams that they bring, or for matter, in the dreams that we have about them. Masud Khan wrote eloquently about the changing use of dreams in psychoanalytic practice (1976, 325). Here he speaks of the way that "a person can hide her true self behind the most bizarre psychopathology, but given the right holding environment the untried capacities can begin to function with amazing intactness and efficiency."

This talk explores the analytic group as an ideal holding environment in which the wishes and fears that find masked expression in dreams can be brought to more conscious expression. Peter Schlachet (1992) and others have explored the specific ways that groups elicit and use dreams. I will address the use of the dream in group therapy from the point of view of its value to the dreamer, to the group-as-a-whole, and as a source of counter-transference information to the leader as well.

Let me offer a dream of one patient in a therapy group. Mr. A. is a 48-year-old single White man who was a member of this group for about 3 years, and for the first time ever, he came in and spontaneously announced that he had had the following dream:

I am sailing alone, in a large, gray, refurbished World War II vessel . . . maybe a former destroyer. It's a bit battered, but it has been mended and painted, and it's in pretty good shape after all. I am pulling into a safe harbor. All of a sudden, I notice there are some sailboats approaching, and I am very worried that they will not see me, and tack across my bow, too close to be safe. Or, if they do see me, they will jeer at the battered ship that has no place in a sailboat race. In either case, I get more and more agitated. Then I notice that nearby and a bit behind me is a small boat, maybe a tugboat. It's a friendly little boat, and I'm pleased to see it there. It makes me smile, and I feel peaceful again, and somehow proud of this old ship. We've been through some hard times together, and it has held up well over the years.

It should be said that the dreamer was a very isolated man with impressive narcissistic problems, and who had spent many an agonizing meeting coming to grips with the idea that the other members of the group might have input with one another that could be trusted. He looked to the leader, who was also treating him individually twice a week, and saw only her coldness in the group, which he contrasted to the warmth that he tended to feel in the individual hours. This dream followed the leader's return from a 2-week absence in the summer.

The Dreamer and the Dream

Again quoting from Masud Kahn, "The dream still provides us with the most condensed, vivid and complex specimens of the conflictual intrapsychic, intersystemic, as well as the interpersonal experiences in any given individual" (p. 328). If so, then let's look at this dream from the point of view of those dimensions for our patient.

This very shame-prone man had been resolutely positive about his experience in the group when the others would ask him about his relative lack of any real material about himself. He tended to be helpful to others, issuing advice or criticism in equal measure, but had remained pretty guarded. His dream led to associations on his part that began to hint at his terror of the others, and his vulnerability:

"Just because it's old and repaired doesn't mean it isn't as desirable."

"WW2 was the only good war."

"My father was in the navy, and nearly got shot out of the water by subs."

"Only that the little boat seems to be following close by, and the two boats seem to go together somehow. It all feels pretty safe. There are no other people that I can see on any of the boats."

Mr. A's access to his unconscious fears and wishes emerged in this dream and we are left to wonder what allowed this deeper level of participation in his unconscious life. It seems likely that the contagion and amplification in the group-as-a-whole allowed him to sail in the same waters with the others, and to finally own some negative transference toward the therapist, which he had heretofore denied almost completely. During her prior absences, he had no awareness of concern and felt only relief that he had some "time off." The current awareness of anxiety on his part was split off in the group, with the negative transference directed more explicitly toward the other slicker sailboats, and an attempt to protect his idealizing transference toward the leader. Once put into words, he heard his associations to his father nearly being shot out of the water, and felt that in the break he had been shot out of the group and the individual situation. The comforting presence of the tugboat hints at his beginning awareness of safety in numbers, although he can still not see any faces on those boats. The father shot out of the water implies some of his wish/fear that the leader would meet a similar fate, and his next association is again one of peacefulness. As various members of the group associated to his dream, he came to see reflected in their mirrored associations aspects of himself about which he had been quite blind. For example, one member associated to his own near drowning experience in camp, and at how dependent he was on his fellow campers to rescue him. When he told his mother about this, she derided him for not having taken all his earlier swimming lessons seriously enough. Another member associated to the Titanic, and to the folly of the narcissistic captain; she was a person who regularly accused the patient of being narcissistic and stuck-up in the group. Yet another woman spoke of the horror-movie quality of not seeing any humans on the other boats, and of how she always felt very alone, especially in the group. Finally, a new member said he did not ever expect to dream, given how revealing a dream could be for the dreamer, and said how impressed he was about the dreamer's openness, which was not being appreciated by the others. All these personal reflections helped the dreamer to see the complexity of his feelings, and to feel intrigued by his internal life. At the same time, he longed for the safety of the individual hours, but had to admit that the crescendo of affect in this moment was more intense than he had ever experienced in his treatment.

The Dream and the Group-as-a-Whole

The relative health of a group culture is characterized by the flexibility of roles and the availability to the ego of the range and complexity of intrapsychic impulses and interpersonal wishes and desires of its members. This group consisted of members whose primary defenses were more narcissistic in nature, and who tended to see the world in black and white. Grandiosity and a fragile empathic capacity characterized their interactions; all were very successful in the world of work, and so found their defenses amply rewarded in terms of status and money. This was certainly true for Mr. A. as well.

Their shared pain centered on the bleakness of their personal lives and their tendency to deep depression and depletion when real or imagined failures became visible to them or, worse still, to others in their surround. What replaced individual capacity for empathy was the cohesion and shared unconscious communications in the group-as-a-whole.

The uncanny attunement that Schlachet referred to is a powerful force for expanding the benefits of any individual's dream and intensifying the work of the whole group. For example, this group of quite narcissistic people had tended to sit in separate sailboats, so to speak, and indeed, those boats did sometime seem impersonal and empty. The group tended to "split their vote" about the value of the leader, and indeed of the whole group experience. Two members regularly made reference to the leader's quiet, saying, "We might as well just have an empty chair there for all you do to help us." Mr. A's dream led to a deepening awareness of the shared longing for rescue, and of their tendency to cut each other off at the pass, in order to claim group time. The competition visible in Mr. A's dream allowed for a more conscious reflection of the hunger and rivalry among many members in the group. Some had begun to scapegoat Mr. A. for his endless idealization of the leader while they maintained a more solidly negative one; the associations to this dream began to modulate the perception of the leader and of one another as all being in the same boat, as one member kept saying.

Put another way, the split off projective-identifications among the members of the group were slowly challenged in the relative safety of the dream material, since the dream allows for a partial disowning of impulses that are not yet available to the patients' conscious ego. "It's only a dream" allows the devil his voice, as one member said, and who could really censor or control or be responsible for a dream since the devil never sleeps?

The Dream and the Group Leader

The group leader has the advantage and the challenge of dealing with all the vectors of transference in the group toward her, as well as toward others and toward the group-as-a-whole. Multiple transferences of course involve multiple countertransferences, all operating to simultaneously bombard the leader's ego and to catalyze her own internal conflicts, interpersonal biases, and so forth. She needs all the help she can get, and the dream material in the group is invaluable source of increased ego awareness in the clinical role. For example, as she listened to Mr. A's dream she had the follow silent but powerful associations:

"Finally, the glacier is melting."

"Say, how do I feel about being Tugboat Annie?"

"I love to sail. Can he know it? Do I want him to know it? To invade a source of such pleasure for me? To accompany me in my fantasy?"

"So how come he can dream for the group, but only very rarely in the individual treatment?"

"Am I doing things to support his idealization, and to block the group's more positive feelings for me and for each other?"

The therapist had been aware for some time that she was worried about Mr. A's tendency toward depression, and feared his oceanic fantasies as indicative of some danger for him. He drank too much, and spoke of watering down his drinks in an effort to drink less. The emergence of this dream in the group was very reassuring in that he finally was finding a life raft in the relationships in the group. She was not his sole source of human contact and support, as she had felt through most of his treatment.

In addition, this group of narcissistic patients generated object hunger in the leader, something of which she was aware, but sometimes forgot that she was also containing the tremendous object hunger of all the members sitting in the room. Their status in the world stimulated some envy and admiration in her at times— some had MacArthur grants, one was a Nobel laureate. The images of Mr. A's empty sailboats, however magnificent they looked, served as a poignant reminder of the reality of their internal states. She was helped to realign more forcefully and empathically on the side of their internal experience and to continue to deepen the work. She woke from a dream of her own soon thereafter thinking about the "belly of the whale," and smiled at the awareness of her wishes/fears of incorporating and being eaten by this group.

Considerations of Technique

Freud cautioned against the pursuit of the dream as a hermeneutic fetish. His caution is well taken in groups where the pursuit of dreams can constitute a resistance as much as it may be a source of rich access to unconscious material. The distributed transferences and the tendency to scapegoat in groups call for a more conscious attention to techniques for working with dreams in groups.

I have found it useful to work in the following way as much as the group process allows without unduly stultifying the group interactions:

- The dreamer is given the space to relate the dream with as little interruption as possible.
- The dreamer is asked whether his dream may be used as a group-wide dream.
- Assuming the dreamer can bear to share "ownership" of his dream, and not until then, other members are invited for their personal associations to the dream.
- Members are encouraged to avoid interpreting the dreamer's dream for him, which can result in 8 people feeling free to analyze the dreamer from a hidden place. Instead all are encouraged to act as though the dream were their own, and associate at will.
- The dreamer is then invited to retell his dream with any details that were omitted or forgotten the first time around.

- The leader is free always to interpret, clarify, and otherwise deepen the work around the dream for the all the members.
- At that point, the group is free to continue the group interactions spontaneously as usual. The above are offered as guidelines and not to be taken as strict rules, in any sense. In dream analysis as in anything else, the art of the work is in the leader's and the groups' sense of staying in synchrony with the alliance and the needs of that particular set of people.

In summary, I want to say that working with dreams in group therapy leads to a complex and rich tapestry that greatly enlivens the work and deepens the waters for all concerned. To stay with my patient's dream metaphor, there is nothing as fine as a sailboat regatta on a warm summer day, in or outside the group room.

References

Khan, M. (1976). The changing use of dreams in psychoanalytic practice: In search of the dreaming experience. *International Journal of Psychoanalysis, 57*: 325.

Schlachet, P. (1972). The dream in group therapy: A reappraisal of unconscious processes in groups. *Group, 16*(4).

Self Psychology in Group Psychotherapy

Self psychology, as originated by Heinz Kohut in the early 1970s, broke the mold on the experience-distant aspect of psychoanalysis. The "blank screen" was being challenged by Kohut and others as too remote and too distant from the struggling patient. Kohut emphasized an empathetic connection between the analyst and the patient. Heinz Kohut's work and writings truly revolutionized the practice of psychoanalysis; there was a shift in the "analytic attitude." This chapter explores the evolution of self psychology as it applies to group psychotherapy. Because self psychology is a newer theory, we are fortunate to have some of the pioneers who developed the theory for groups on our faculty, as well as among our guest presenters. The papers presented in this chapter begin with an introduction to self psychology by Dr. Sy Rubenfeld, the founding director of the National Group Psychotherapy Institute. A paper by Dr. Rosemary Segalla follows, where she fully explores the development of self psychology as a theoretical perspective for group psychotherapy. Dr. Segalla cites the work of notable contributors in the development of the theory such as Dr. Joseph Lichtenburg and Dr. Irene Harwood, both presenters at our self psychology weekends. Dr. Harwood's paper "Toward Optimum Group Placement From the Perspective of the Self or Self-Experience" is a seminal paper in the field, in which she clearly spells out the necessity to use our understanding of the patient's needs and level of development in selecting a group for them. At the conclusion, there are two application papers by Mary Dluhy: one on working with anger in group therapy and the other on working with intersubjectivity.

Mary Dluhy

A Brief Introduction to Self Psychology

SY RUBENFELD

Self psychology began in the work of its originator Heinz Kohut as a special theory of narcissistic disorders and their treatability in a psychoanalytic frame, but has evolved into what some of its adherents consider a broadly new paradigm of treatment. This has an interesting parallel to my mind with the way American therapists became familiar with some of the processes crucial to broad-based object relations thinking, such as splitting, projection, projective identification, and denial, first as properties of special pathological states like borderline conditions, through Kernberg's and Masterson's writings in the 1970s. What is introduced to understand and treat what was previously thought to be untreatable gains wide currency as we apply it to ourselves and our patients.

It has been rightly said that Kohut failed to honor his debt to Winnicott's ideas about self developing in the holding context of good-enough mothering. But Kohut became convinced, based on his clinical experience, that before other problems, as an analyst working within a classical drive/structure theory, he had to repair narcissistic damage and that it could be done psychoanalytically; to him that meant that narcissistic transferences could be formed and resolved.

Paralleling the idea that an authentic self is cultivated by the sensitive facilitation of a good-enough mother, self psychology as developed by Kohut and his followers propounds the following as some of its main ideas: To develop a strong, vital, and cohesive self, a child must form attachment to parent figures who adequately perform certain specific functions as a certain kind of object called selfobjects. There is a developmental line from infantile grandiosity to a relatively stable self-esteem. Through their affirming *mirroring* of a child's being and qualities, his selfobjects facilitate this growth. A child will also *idealize* a parenting figure as an externalization of his early omnipotence.

Optimally this idealized other enables the child to internalize reasonable standards and values by which to judge his accomplishments and set his goals. Other important self-object functions are providing *twinship* or alter ego experiences (i.e., that another is like oneself, found with a sib or someone like H. S. Sullivan's chum) and providing an empathic function for protecting and maturing adversarial needs, such as healthy competitiveness and aggressivity. Recognition of this by self psychologists contradicts those who might think that self psychology is just psychic handholding, or that it's only what any tactful therapist might do anyway.

Especially important for group therapy is the notion that persons continue to need a responsiveness in others throughout their lives to support these operations of the self. Persons can and do perform *reciprocal* selfobject functions for one another (much like Yalom's parable about the rabbi who is shown the difference between heaven and hell). As Dr. Rosemary Segalla of our Group Therapy Faculty and her associates have shown in their writing, multiple selfobject functions may be performed by cotherapists and other group members. The group therapist's modeling of empathic attunement is like yeast or starter dough, transmitted by members' identification into the culture and mores of the group.

Parenting figures may significantly fail in these selfobject functions through insensitive neglect, continual interference, demandingness, or repressive criticalness. (Again, these are like Winnicott's maternal impingement). When they do, damage to the self occurs. The person is susceptible thereafter to disintegrative feelings of inferiority, unacceptability, failure, envy, helpless frustration. A person may distance himself from others to avoid wounded rage. He may resort to anxious or denied avoidance of anticipated selfobject failure by others who become important, like his therapist. Resistances in therapy can be these same self-protective reactions. Self psychology is a deficit theory insofar as it asserts that these vulnerabilities in the self precede conflict developmentally and causally and therefore should take precedence therapeutically. Oedipal conflict, for instance, in feelings of rivalry or jealousy, may have something to do with parents' failures to tune in empathically on the child's healthy competitiveness and assertiveness to help him or her to sustain these capacities. Or, to put it in object relations terms, the Oedipus complex is a triangle experienced in the schizoid-paranoid mode, that a person might be stuck with and in as a result of phase-appropriate self-object functioning. A major distinction in treatment approach is that the therapist must attend to and repair these self deficits first, or otherwise run the risk of causing the patient to feel judged, or misjudged, and threatened by conflict-oriented interpretations.

A patient in resistance attempts to avoid further injury to his self. It is one thing for a patient to imagine that the other is indifferent or hostile. That reflects the patient's internalized bad part objects. It is another matter when he does not imagine that the other is capable of joining him empathically. This expresses the limitations or narcissistic demands he expects to find in the person of the therapist or another group member.

In too much of a nutshell, the theory of treatment here calls for a primary empathic stance that provides an optimal responsiveness to the selfobject needs of the patient. The therapist expects to be experienced as failing in these functions, inevitably, sooner or later; his/her empathic involvement is ready to assist the patient to identify where he/she felt misunderstood. Self-psychological theory of therapeutic effect concentrates on this break in empathic involvement as experienced by the patient. The therapist wants to identify it, explain it as such, and interpret its significance in terms of the patient's childhood experience.

Therapeutic benefit derives not just from optimizing on the patient's frustrations with the therapist but on providing the empathic mirroring or functioning as an approachable ideal object. Stolorow and his colleagues have written the maximum therapeutic benefit occurs in the climate of understanding intersubjectivity that therapist and patient create together. Dr. Segalla and her associates have stated that group is a much more powerful venue than individual for self-psychological repair and working through, and I tend to agree.

Dr. Skolnick in a published paper of his points out a comment of Bion's, after he stopped working with groups, that there can be no understanding without love; love of the group and by the group means the holding and facilitating climate generated by many selves in continually deepening intersubjectivity. It is very noteworthy that Dr. Giraldo works from an object relations perspective, as we have seen, and yet in his kindness and tact I thought I saw how much of a good-enough group mother a good group therapist and his members can be. I will try to indicate some of these actions from mostly a self-psychological standpoint. Though I don't consider myself a self psychologist in my work, as you will see in some of my comments about the group, I consider self psychology an invaluable contribution to the work. I believe that ultimately self-psychology is a theory of the self as subject and not as object, and therapeutically explores ways of joining with the self as subject. I recently heard Dr. John Dluhy of our faculty say that he views the selfobject as a person who is experienced as knowing the uniqueness of the subject person. Self psychology may really be about creating openings for the true self of Winnicott, Fairbairn, and Guntrip to emerge. From the standpoint of an existential humanism, self psychology enables the self to be the agent of an authentic whole person.

Beyond the Dyad

An Evolving Theory of Group Psychotherapy

ROSEMARY A. SEGALLA

The long and varied history of theory development in group psychotherapy, and its clinical application, has in many ways mirrored the vicissitudes of theory development in psychoanalysis and the individual psychotherapies. It has been both applauded as a revolutionary approach to the treatment of emotional disorders and condemned as a technique that endangers the psychological health of the individual. Even a cursory survey of the vast body of literature on group psychotherapy could cause one to question the necessity of adding still another perspective. And yet in an age of rapid development of relational perspectives in psychoanalysis and psychotherapy it seems remiss not to extend the dialogue to include group psychotherapy.

Despite the recent paradigm shifts within modern psychoanalysis, group treatment remains a shadowy and somewhat disregarded mode of treatment. I have been curious about its absence from the discussions of relationalists, intersubjectivists, and others who clearly view psychoanalysis as the study of "people's experiences and the meaning of experiences" (Galatzer-Levy and Cohler, 1993, p. 341). These authors operating from an open system perspective state that "people seek increasingly sophisticated interdependence and use others to enhance self-affirmation at all times, but especially during times of distress and psychological growth" (p. 347). They go on to state that "the goal of psychological intervention ought to be to assist the analyzing to obtain satisfaction from reliance on others and receive greater satisfaction and comfort from a continuing use of others across the course of life" (p. 347). I suggest that group treatment is a natural extension of an individual analysis and a modality especially well suited to promote the growth necessary to cope effectively with life's many complex endeavors. If one accepts the basic premise that "the self cannot be understood apart from life with others" (p. 358), then we can be curious about the relative inattention that the group treatment modality has received from the psychoanalytic community, especially that part of the community that is currently so warmly embracing relational and intersubjective perspectives. Perhaps this reflects an unconscious continued emphasis on "self-reliant individual independence" and the persistence of the "unfounded assumption that separation and independence are normative" (p. 359). A group offers us vital information about the impact and necessity of essential others, information that is not fully available in the traditional psychoanalytic dyad.

In this presentation I will explore the evolution of my own theory of group psychotherapy as it has been formed by my experiences as a group therapist and by my role on the faculty of a group *psychotherapy* institute. The discussion will be from a perspective reflective of the selfobject, multiple selfobject, intersubjectivity, motivational systems, and the groupobject.

Kohut's Influence

Because Kohut developed his theory from clinical experiences with psychoanalytic patients, he did not expand it beyond a dyadic model *of* treatment. His paper, "Creativeness, Charisma, Group Psychotherapy" (1976), however captures his awareness of, and sensitivity to, group issues. He suggested that just as there is an individual "self," there is a "group self." He viewed the study of group phenomena as essential, recognizing that all aspects of group, from its formation through its "oscillations between group fragmentation and reintegration," were significant. He was abundantly clear about our continuous engagement with the other and in his final book *How Does Analysis Cure* (1994) he offers his view about selfobject relatedness which is basic to self psychologically oriented group work. He states, "Self psychology holds that the self-selfobject relationships form the essence of psychological life from birth to death, that a move from dependence to independence in the psychological sphere is no more possible than a corresponding move from a life dependent on oxygen to a life independent of it in the biological sphere" (p. 47).

In my early writing on group therapy (1985) I presented my ideas from a strictly Kohutian perspective. In that early paper I emphasized the selfobject experiences of the individual group members, focusing on the expansion of selfobject experiences in a cotherapy, combined treatment model. I postulated that group members had ample opportunities to have selfobject experiences that reinforced those found in the individual treatment. I further suggested that the group itself develops the need for selfobjects and that just as transferences developed in the individual, they develop in the group. I state the following:

> I find clear examples of mirroring, idealizing and alter ego transferences at play in the group-as-a-whole. These group level reactions require the same process of *understanding* and *explaining* in order for the group

to grow in cohesiveness and toward mature selfobject functions. So, in addition to thinking of transmuting internalizations on the level of the individual, we can consider that this happens on the group level as well. How would this be manifested and commented upon? The level of complexity of such a situation is immediately apparent. (1985, p. 8)

Expanding the selfobject to a multiple selfobject concept (Harwood, 1986; Segalla, Silvers, Wine & Pillsbury, 1988) was an obvious next step. Harwood (1986) suggests that "Those in related fields of child development, psychoanalysis, and social research need to understand the positive and negative conditions and effects of multiple or extended selfobject experience upon the evolving self structure as well as the intersubjective context in which interaction takes place" (p. 291). She emphasizes the need for "many different selfobject functions" (p. 295). Segalla et al., unaware of Harwood's conclusions, came to a very similar perspective:

The multiple selfobject environment more accurately reproduces the early experiences of most of us. It dramatically recreates the move from one caretaker to several and so on to such settings as preschool, school, and jobs. By creating this complex group environment, we are creating a therapeutic environment in which these additional factors can be best addressed. One of the most significant aspects of viewing groups as multiple selfobject experiences, is that it opens to sharper scrutiny relationships with other important people such as siblings, hired caretakers, school teachers, grandparents, etc. who in fact may have provided significant experiences for patients. It may also shed light on those situations in which it seems remarkable that a person has done as well as they have considering the apparently major deficits present in their primary caretaker. (1988, p. 6)

We emphasized accessing existing aspects of the self unavailable in the selfobject transferences of individual treatment and postulated that the addition of group treatment broadened and deepened our access to disturbances of the self. We likened the experience of moving from individual to group treatment as a move from considering the impact of the primary caregiver to that of the whole family system (including other caregivers and cultural institutions such as churches and schools). As a result of this thinking a multiple selfobject model was formulated. In this model the cotherapists, along with group members, supply multiple selfobject functions for each other. Because of this shift, the notion of what is healing was expanded to include the rich complexity of dyadic, subgroup, and group-as-a-whole interactions operating simultaneously. The original theoretical thinking was based on a point made by Kohut in *How Does Analysis Cure?* He said,

In a properly conducted analysis, that is, an analysis that does not block the spontaneous unfolding of the transferences, the basic and pivotal selfobject transference that ultimately establishes itself will frequently be organized around the less traumatic aspect of the selfobject parents. (1984, p. 206)

Thus, Kohut suggested that in the development of compensatory structures, the person has turned away from a part of the self which was not growth producing and that attempting to address this aspect of the self can result in an unnecessary regression that would ultimately not be curative.

What then becomes of these more damaged aspects of self? It was at this point that we began to speculate about why, when we placed someone in a group who had a long and rather successful individual treatment, did we see new behaviors that often appeared to be regressive throwbacks to earlier times. These were patterns that were not seen or experienced in the more empathically immersed individual treatment, but were problematic interactions that might have been described by the patient as occurring in other relationships or in other settings. We found that the sensitivity and reactivity of the patient in group highlighted aspects of the self that were sometimes referenced in individual treatment but were never manifested prior to entry into group therapy. We observed that while it was threatening for group members to experience aspects of the self that they had not explored in their individual work, it ultimately created an expanded flexibility of functioning.

In developing the multiple selfobject model, we extend Kohut's definition of the healing power of a therapeutic relationship to include not only the second therapist but also the other group members. That is, we found that the process of empathic engagement by the therapists with a group member(s), or the whole group, was gradually adopted by the members themselves and became a part of group culture. Instead of reacting primarily out of their own individual needs, they were gradually able to engage at the level of empathic inquiry and in doing so acquired the skills needed to work through empathic ruptures with each other. As the group develops, this process among members dominates the sessions, with the therapists gradually moving into a background position as the patients learn to work more effectively with each other.

The process of learning to be optimally responsive (Bacal, 1985) to each other, working through empathic ruptures and being affectively engaged promotes healthy functioning. We suggested that experiences in group therapy are most readily transferable to the larger world, providing the patient with an expanded capacity to deal with the multiple realities encountered in daily life. This leads to greater flexibility and, therefore, the possibility of having selfobject experiences as well as fostering the capacity to provide selfobject experiences to others. In leaving the protected environment in which a therapist focuses her full attention on the relationship with one person, a group provides the possibility of activating a process that allows the patient to be both affectively aware of their own wishes and needs as well as engaging in an active process of learning about how they are viewed and how they view others.

We have found that the well established selfobject transference with the therapist, as well as the interplay between individual and group treatment, insures opportunities to work through potentially traumatic experiences. This is most apparent when someone is placed directly into a group without the intervening modulating experience of individual treatment. This circumstance seems to result in a greater possibility of empathic rupture and often leads to an early departure from group.

We also came to view engagement among members as selfobject *transferences* and saw the exploration of these transferences as a primary curative factor. This view differs from Wolf (1988) who distinguished between selfobject *experiences* and selfobject *transferences* with the latter occurring *only* with the therapist. We suggested that the opportunity to establish and work through selfobject transferences among group members, under the guidance of the group therapists, provides a unique opportunity to heal aspects of the self unaddressed in individual treatment. The group setting is unique in its ability to reactivate early experiences that have remained more or less unconscious in the dyadic treatment. A brief case example should help illustrate these points.

Larry was a high-functioning man in his late 30s who was doing an important piece of work in his individual treatment. He was a robust and warm person who, despite a significant depression, managed to maintain himself in a relationship and a responsible job. His idealized selfobject transference to me seemed to address unmet developmental needs with both parents. At the point he entered group after 4 years of individual treatment, he was grappling with his disappointment in his marriage and in himself for being unable to complete and publish a book. In the group, I very was surprised by the significant difficulty this lively man had in finding his voice. He rarely spoke and when he did, it was not sufficiently engaging for the group to attend to him so the discussion would shift to other members. He would look discouraged briefly, but then in a good-humored way become engaged. The repetition of this pattern and the ultimate meaning we were able to get from it was an important and central part of his work. The emergence of this aspect of Larry's self was significantly absent in his individual work prior to his entry into group. In his sessions with me, he was active and curious, raising issues spontaneously. His ability to be both exploratory and assertive (Lichtenberg, 1989) seemed to make him a good candidate for group. When he entered group I was unprepared for this apparent willingness to put aside his own subjective self, a self that was clearly present in his twice-weekly individual sessions.

His difficulty seemed to be indicative of a family dynamic as well as a father/son dyadic bond that we had discussed in individual therapy, but had never been available for us to work through transferentially. The inhibition he exhibited in group was useful in supplying information as to why he was unable to advance in his chosen profession and why his voice seemed so effectively silenced in his marriage. The information and emotions that emerged in the group experience allowed us to explore these issues in depth, and greatly aided him in moving forward in his life.

Intersubjectivity

Like the growth of ideas that has continued to create a lively dialogue within self psychology, group therapists have been impacted by the move within psychoanalysis toward a relational perspective. Some aspects of this were foreshadowed by Kohut when he wrote about the "impact of the observer on the observed" (1959). Stolorow and Atwood (1992) state: "Self experience is always organized within a constitutive intersubjective context and is shaped at every point in development by the intersubjective system in which it crystallizes" (p. 17). They credit Beebe and Lachmann's (1988) infant research and their conceptualization of a system of reciprocal mutual influence, stating that "the concept of an intersubjective system brings to focus both the individual's world of inner experience and its embeddedness with other worlds in a continual flow or reciprocal mutual influence. In this vision, the gap between the intrapsychic and interpersonal realms is closed" (1992, p. 18).

One implication of the intersubjective perspective for group treatment is the change in the view of empathic ruptures. Stolorow et al. (1992) redefine them as "intractable repetitive transferences" resulting from the interface of the patient's problems with the therapist's issues, preventing the therapist from being optimally responsive to the patient's affective state. This reflects their view that the individual's selfobject needs exist alongside conflictual resistive needs. These two positions constitute a bipolar model viewed as more encompassing than simply attending to selfobject issues. This is particularly important in group treatment, where an overemphasis on either pole, selfobject or conflictual/resistive, leaves a considerable gap in understanding of group phenomena.

Indeed, group therapists have been negative about self psychology because they viewed the emphasis on selfobject functioning as ignoring much of the aggressive aspects of the self manifested in group therapy. Several other points have been made: Silvers (1998), pointing to the value inherent in expanding the experiential field, states: "Adding a group experience to an ongoing individual treatment expands the therapeutic intersubjective field, exposing patients to a wider range of selfobject and conflictual, repetitive and resistive transference phenomena. The presence of the second therapist in the cotherapy model stimulates transference material concerning the other (second) parent that does not emerge in the individual treatment or when there is a single therapist" (pp. 136–137). Shapiro (1998), emphasizing twinship selfobject experience, states: "Group therapy provides many opportunities for intersubjective exploration and to move patients from archaic to mature twinship experiences. The twinship or alterego experience is the foundation of cohesiveness in group therapy and may be more basic to the human condition than the other selfobject experience" (p. 56). Harwood (1998) points to the growth that results from a group therapist's ability to assist the group members in clarifying experience and *constructing* meanings from the selfobject, as well as conflictual, repetitive, and resistive transferences at play in the group.

Paparo and Nebbiosi (1998) see the two dimensions of the transference proposed by Stolorow and Atwood as useful in understanding "the complex transference dimension of the group that . . . is characterized by the fact that *repetitive and selfobject transferences occur simultaneously,* By this we mean that while a member can experience a repetitive transference (to the analyst) he can experience a selfobject transference at the same (to the group-as-a-whole or to another member). In this last case, the group analyst should be able to handle both of the dimensions of transference that can occur at different levels" (pp. 73–74).

My own perspective (as well as that of Silvers, 1998) is that this intersubjective model is also salient when considering trauma and the potential for its escalation in a group setting. In their exploration of trauma, Stolorow and Atwood suggest that "painful or frightening affect becomes traumatic when the requisite attuned responsiveness that the child needs from the surround to assist in its tolerance, *containment,* modulation and alleviation is absent" (1992, p. 53). We have found that the number and complexity of interactions in a group make it unlikely that all traumatic experiences will be addressed within the group. Therefore we have continued to work from a combined individual and group treatment model. This model provides some assurance that injuries, if unaddressed or missed in the group context, will be explored in the individual therapy.

A further issue that is particularly important in considering the placement of a patient in a group is the potential for the reenactment of a core problem related to the development of the self. That is, if the patient has not resolved her own conflict around her sense of self, then:

> A fundamental psychic conflict . . . becomes established between the requirement that one's developmental course must conform to the emotional needs of caregivers and the inner imperative that its evolution be firmly rooted in a vitalizing affective core of one's own. As one of several possible outcomes of this basic conflict, the child may be compelled to abandon or severely compromise central affective strivings in order to maintain indispensable ties. (Stolorow and Atwood, p. 79)

Brandchaft (1991, 1998) describes this as pathological accommodation. It is not difficult to think of group patients who seem only too willing to accommodate to the group culture, leaving their own needs unaddressed and thereby reactivating a pathological process from childhood. This can occur despite a good individual treatment that has reinforced self development.

A recent example of this was Jack, who was placed in a long-term group because of his difficulties in intimate relationships. In his individual sessions he was emotionally responsive and able to address his fears of the therapist's perceived requirement—that he behave himself by agreeing with whatever she said. The therapist was also acutely aware of his sensitivity to her slightest expression and his readiness to accommodate to subtle messages she might convey. The individual sessions explored these issues and this resulted in a gradual understanding of what, in the interplay with the therapist, had led him to believe that there was a required way of being. The work was intense but rewarding, and Jack seemed a good candidate for group therapy, primarily because despite his improvement, he continued to have difficulty in maintaining relationships. His entry into the group went smoothly, and his capacity to engage group members was initially well received. Gradually, however, as he continued over several weeks to raise the affective ante of the group, the members began to react by lecturing, scolding, and withdrawing from him. Both therapists explored the group members' responses to Jack, as well as his responses to them. Various dyadic interactions emerged and were explored intersubjectively from the members' perspectives.

What gradually unfolded however was a silencing of Jack, and acquiescence on his part. What was now being reactivated in the group was the very process that Jack frequently discussed in his individual sessions. Working with him in both individual and group, it became clear that he had been either ignored or fawned over by his mother. When he was a "good boy," she was loving; when he was "bad," she was cold and rageful. Jack's primary task was to provide selfobject experiences for this severely damaged woman. Having this dynamic enacted in group helped Jack more fully understand the cost of accommodation to his mother's excessive and unpredictable emotional demands. The group experience also helped Jack begin to see how he was unable to modulate himself in his relationships with women. He either accommodated to the other, losing a sense of his own self, or he reacted without any sense of the other, behaving in a self-absorbed manner. This issue was explored over and over as its various permutations were enacted in the group.

As part of the group process, the members come to appreciate their "interacting subjectivities." They see that any engagement must be considered from the perspective of each member. The idea of interacting subjectivities is useful in eliminating group tendencies to polarize into good guy–bad guy, victim-victimizer. What emerges is a group culture in which people consider their own responses and reactions to those of other group members, as well as those of the therapists, eliminating the need to blame, and opening an arena where reactions can be explored.

Considering the group from an intersubjective perspective can be a daunting, but useful task. It encourages the group to work in the moment and makes resistances and defenses as interesting to the members and therapists as full cooperation. Disruptions are viewed as inevitable, but workable. The decrease in primary emphasis on selfobject experiences in fact increases the therapist's sensitivity to conflictual material, encouraging a broader affective range. It has proved to be an approach that takes full advantage of the here and now of the group. This perspective also encourages the therapist to consider their own reactions to a variety of group events in which their own reactions may be disruptive to group process (Segalla, 1997).

Motivational Systems

Despite Kohut's reference to group self and the work of the intersubjectivists there have been few efforts by theoreticians to see group as a natural extension of the theorizing about the self-psychological dyad. Writers in this area do not fully explore the implications of our embeddedness in familial and social contexts. Lichtenberg, however, is an exception. In his book *Psychoanalysis and Motivation* (1989) he addresses this issue directly. While his primary emphasis is on the individual he also acknowledges the inherent need for affiliation. This recognition of an environment beyond a dyadic encounter is basic to his conceptualization of five motivational systems.

Five Motivational Systems and Group Therapy

In *Psychoanalysis and Motivation* (1989), Lichtenberg suggests five motivational systems inherent in the individual that operate to regulate and fill basic needs. These are:

> (1) the need for psychic regulation of physiological requirements, (2) the need for attachment and later affiliation, (3) the need for exploration and assertion, (4) the need to react aversively through antagonism or withdrawal (or both), and (5) the need for sensual enjoyment and sexual excitement.

In exploring the usefulness of this conceptualization for group treatment, we begin by wondering how these systems might play out in a group. If at every moment in the group a motivational system is dominant for each member and the therapists, we can also assume that the group itself, as well as its various subgroups, is dominated by motivational pulls that shift from moment to moment. My experience is that groups operate primarily from three motivational systems: attachment/affiliation, exploratory/assertion, and aversiveness. The attachment/affiliation system seems to provide the glue needed to keep the group relatively cohesive as it struggles to stay exploratory in the face of aversiveness resulting from the inevitable clashes of incompatible motivations and intersubjective dynamics. Using the motivational system as a background concept to whole group encounters, we can quickly situate ourselves within the group action—tending to the individual, the dyad, and the whole group. So, for example, if one therapist is working with a member or aiding a subgroup in a particular exploration, the second therapist can be monitoring the affective and attentional atmosphere of the whole group. Does the exploratory motivational system appear to be dominant for the other members, or are there indications that members are reacting aversively by withdrawal?

These shifts in motivational dominance are informed by affective reactions both in the individual and the whole group. An example of this is a recent experience Allen had in group. Unlike his usual stance of relative quiet, Allen spoke out in the group about the tardiness of some members. Since he so rarely raised his voice in any criticism of group members, his reaction caught everyone's attention. The group, which had begun the session in an affiliative mode, shifted to an exploratory mode with Allen. This focus led to more and more confusion for Allen. He was unable, despite the fact that he is a very articulate person, to express his feelings. The group seemed equally frustrated by Allen's inability to shift out of an aversive withdrawal and engage with them. The group's frustration resulted in their own withdrawal and the group-as-a-whole was left with a sense of confusion. Although Allen was unable to move into an exploratory mode with the group he came for his individual session, with written notes about his reactions to the previous group. He spent the individual hour trying to make sense of his aversive withdrawal in reaction to the exploratory focus of the group. While the individual session calmed him, it also gave him some insights as to why he was so stymied by the group's interest in his reaction and helped him understand how he sidestepped their interest when it felt too intrusive. His written notes capture his ability to be exploratory and they highlight the developmental importance of the individual therapy where a secure and tested attachment allows him to remain in an exploratory mode long enough to process his reactions to group. This illustrates how a patient attempts to negotiate their way through individual and group therapy, using the relatively secure and tested attachment to the individual therapist to modulate the experiences within the less secure affiliation of the group.

Model Scenes

Model scenes, a formalization of experiences that are a regular part of psychoanalytic treatment, can be usefully expanded to group treatment where affective reactions by group members are the basis of much of the group intercourse. Lichtenberg et al. (1989) state: "They (model scenes) draw on the fundamental inclination of analyst and analysand to organize experience in terms of events or episodes. Because of the clinical purpose they serve, the events selected are those amplified by an affective response triggered when the needs of a motivational system are met or more likely for the analysis, unmet" (p. 25).

The authors see model scenes as providing information about both content and process. The content is the story, or as they call it, the scene, while the process tends to the patient's state of mind, explored in the empathic, intersubjective engagement with the therapist. The usefulness of model scenes is immediately apparent in group where the narrative flow is rich and continuous. Often a model scene will emerge when there has been a disruption of some kind, either for a member, a subgroup, or the entire group. The work on the model scene can bring a kind of cohesion to the group as it struggles to understand a particular experience. Additionally, there can be an interplay between individual and group treatment in that a model scene constructed in either setting can be readily explored in the group or individual work. The effort of the therapists is to understand the experiences of both the individual and group. An example of a model scene occurred when Ruth complained that she was experiencing the group as a dangerous place to bring her problems. Her outburst came during a group session that had in fact been quite fruitful in its exploration of another member's difficult issue. The group reacted with surprise to Ruth's exclamation and wanted to know more about it. Ruth, in turn, was stunned when she realized that her experience of the session was so different from the other members and the two therapists. She stated that it was her experience that everyone was feeling unsafe. Various group members disagreed and wanted to know more about her reactions. A careful exploration of Ruth's feelings uncovered an issue with which the group was familiar—that is, that Ruth was often scapegoated in her family for saying what was obvious but never acknowledged by other family members. Her willingness to, in her language, call a "spade a spade" endlessly got her in trouble—not just in the family, but everywhere. What emerged in the group work after considerable effort by the members was that for Ruth there was one reality and it was her painful task in life to define and name the reality that others avoided. The group encounter allowed her to expand her own awareness of her early experience and how it had shaped her current reality—one which, in fact, left little room for the realities of others. This model scene became an enduring one for the group and was called upon when needed in working with Ruth or other members. Unlike her experience in her family the group dealt with her subjective difference with considerable interest and curiosity, a reaction that allowed Ruth to explore her own reactiveness nondefensively. Although the familial model scene had originally been verbally reconstructed in the individual therapy, its reemergence in the group caused a powerful affective experience that enabled her to effectively modify a rigidly held reactive stance that had long caused her significant interpersonal difficulties.

Model Scenes Beget Model Scenes

This example of a model scene where the attention is on one member as she worked with the whole group is only one of many other possibilities presented by group treatment. For example, a model scene can emerge in the work between one of the therapists and a group member or the group-as-a-whole. Another possibility is that the group members learn to create model scenes with each other. This can reflect historical experiences of members or it can reflect the history within the group. For example, members will return again and again to particular encounters in the group that seem to provide turning points for members or the whole group. These group model scenes when recalled provide a kind of quick access to strong affective reactions that are part of the group history. The model scene work can be particularly powerful when it occurs between the patient and the "other" therapist. This occurred in a group in which Mark, an individual patient seen by me, constructed a model scene with my cotherapist that was instructive in helping us to understanding his relationship with a withdrawn and disinterested father. The male therapist spontaneously asked Mark about his efforts at job hunting, expressing considerable interest in the possibilities that Mark outlined. Mark suddenly began to cry. As a result of this affective reaction, the two of them began an exploration of Mark's strong emotional response. What became clear was that my cotherapist's interest in Mark activated a painful memory of trying to engage his uninvolved father in helping him choose a college only to have him persist in reading the newspaper. As a result of this rather intensive work with Mark, and the emergence of this model scene, other group members gained access to related material, including their own experiences when they felt the group, and/or the group leaders, was not interested or engaged with them. Thus, in the group, we can say that model scenes beget model scenes, leading the group to work with increasingly more complicated situations with each other and the cotherapists.

Using a Motivational Model

How and where the therapist focuses attention can be an ongoing issue in a group of seven or eight members. This can be particularly difficult in a relatively new group where members are not clear about how they wish to occupy their group space. Working in the foreground/background the therapists can monitor both the individual's motivational dominance as well as the group motivation. A quick moment-to-moment assessment provides information that allows the therapists initially and later, as a group matures, the members themselves to focus on a particular individual or situation. As much as possible this is informed by the within-the-room process and speaks to engagement among members or members and therapists. With two therapists present, one can attend to the whole group motivational system, while the second therapist can attend to the dominant motivational system of a patient member or particular dyad. Such an engagement occurred when Mary was discussing her marriage and move to another state. One therapist was working actively with her around her anxiety that she would be unable to adjust to this new and temporary location, and that her difficulty would have a negative impact on her relationship with her boyfriend. As my cotherapist engaged with her, asking questions and creating a clearer picture of her discomfort, I stayed attuned to the group-as-a-whole and noticed the members becoming progressively more withdrawn as the session progressed. When the opportunity presented itself, I suggested that there seemed to be a mood in the group that was not being expressed. Members began to speak, stating that they felt that despite their interest and engagement earlier in the session, Mary was not responsive. They did not feel listened to and felt that they were being of no help. The group, which had begun in an affiliative engagement with Mary, had moved to an aversive position characterized by withdrawal. There were several comments that suggested that Mary was "whining." The group's flight into silence reflected an aversive withdrawal, which allowed the members to avoid an antagonistic attack, failing to see that their reactions would in fact be useful information for Mary. The first therapist began to explore with Mary what the impact of the withdrawal had been. What became clear was that she did not expect any comfort, and had in fact expected to be rejected by the group because of her departure, though it was temporary. This led to a familial model scene that surrounded her graduation from college and return home. Instead of being welcomed back, she found her large family had essentially written her off. Not feeling accepted back into the home, she moved out with little reaction from her family. The group's earlier efforts to contain and support Mary could not be taken in because, according to Mary, "I know that as soon as I'm gone I'll be forgotten and when I come back in 6 months, it will be too late and I'll never fit back in." The creation of this model scene was very useful for Mary, as well as for the group as a whole. Members found that her resistance to being helped had in fact threatened their sense of agency with each other, an important affiliative task. For her part, Mary began to grasp the extent of her injury within this rejecting family system and how the resulting expectation of disinterest had impacted her first marriage.

Groupobject—Expansion of Selfobject Theory

The conceptualization of a groupobject reflects an effort to further our understanding of group process and its meaning for individual group members, as well as for the whole group. This formulation is an extension of selfobject, multiple selfobject, intersubjectivity and motivational systems theories, which have all been significant in explicating experiences in the therapeutic encounter. In a 1996 paper, I suggested that, just as there exists in the individual the need for healthy selfobject experiences, there is also the need for healthy groupobject experiences. I stated: "The group can be said to possess a set of functions designed to maintain the integrity and cohesiveness of the group self, and a set of functions which provide the group with initiative and goal direction. Along the lines of Stolorow et al., these functions might also serve to organize affective experiences." I suggested that groupobject experiences seem to exist both on the individual and group level and that just as there are selfobject transferences, there are groupobject transferences.

This emphasis on the group is an effort to understand the reality of life within a social system which, almost from birth, expands beyond the infant/caregiver dyad to ever increasing levels of complex engagements in the family, school, peer groups, and so forth of everyday life. Our ability to function within these more complex systems can be understood as being more or less successful based on the availability of healthy selfobject experiences. If, however, we extend our thinking from an individual self to a group self, it suggests the possibility that the group organism operates in many of the same ways as the individual. The groupobject concept can help us gain access to the complexity of group life. Unlike the individual, who may look to external objects to provide selfobject experiences, the group must organize itself so as to provide groupobject experiences to its members from within the group, what I call an intrasubjective experience. This is based on the idea that the human proclivity to group serves a species survival need.

For an individual to relinquish the primacy of vitalizing selfobject experiences in order to be part of a group, she must have group experiences powerful enough to motivate this somewhat dangerous surrender. But it is only by surrendering these needs that the individual can participate in the group's power. The development of the group self begins in the context of the first group, the family; just as there are selfobject experiences that enhance and vitalize the individual, there are groupobject experiences in the family that enhance group functioning. It is these groupobject needs that are most significant in a group therapy and inform us about the quality of earlier group/family/social systems.

Selfobject experiences give the individual the chance to fill missing aspects of the self, groupobject experiences can aid in filling missing aspects of the group. If we accept the premise; demonstrated in infant research (Beebe and Lachmann, 1988), that we are hard-wired for reciprocal mutual responsiveness on the dyadic level, we must consider the postulate that as social animals we are also hard-wired to operate in a mutually responsive manner in groups. And, just as we come to dyadic relationships innately prepared to engage with the other, we come to group experiences (starting with the family) similarly prepared. Thus a primary task of the individual is learning how to function within these larger, more complex systems. The increasing complexity suggests that in learning to function in these group contexts, we must move beyond individual needs and expectations and learn how to function effectively in various groups. This is where the groupobject concept may help us in gaining access to the complexity of the group experience in the small as well as the large group. That is, we can assume that there is an inherent wish to function effectively in a group and beyond the self or dyadic intersubjective experience. I am suggesting that groupobject needs are activated in all groups, and just as we have met with varying degrees of success in getting selfobject needs met, we have varying degrees of success in filling groupobject needs. Our success or failure at the earliest group level, the family, will determine how well we traverse the unknowns of any new group experience, whether in the therapeutic setting or the larger world.

Activating groupobject needs may be powerfully defended against for at least two reasons: One is the fear of the loss of the individual self, and the second is the fear of the loss of the group self. The first fear is related to a dreaded loss of cohesion and the second is the dread of alienation. Failures or trauma at the group self level can lead to the feelings of fragmentation at the individual level and vice versa. Thus, as we speak of dyadic intersubjective experiences, I would like to suggest that there is a dynamic tension between the individual's selfobject needs and their groupobject needs (Segalla, 1997). This tension can be creatively transformed into a process that enhances the growth of both the individual self and the group self. Thus to the extent that someone is successful in having selfobject experiences, she is more available for groupobject experiences. The constant negotiation between individual selfobject experiences and groupobject experiences provides much of the texture of daily life. As we negotiate our way dyadically, we are reassured of our capacity to cope with another, thereby setting the stage for successful engagement on the group level. This suggests that we can predict how well someone may respond in a therapy group in which the emphasis shifts away from the primacy of individual needs to becoming engaged at the group level. The capacity to make this shift is in part the basis of healing on the group level. If the group is responsive to the individual's efforts to engage, we can allow an immersion in the experience. However, if the group is not receptive, then there is a defensive withdrawal and a return to the singleton position (Turquet, 1975). Just as a patient defensively avoids engaging with their therapists because they fear that they will yet again be unable to have successful selfobject experiences, engagement in the group is defensively avoided for fear of failure in having groupobject experiences. Returning to a motivational systems model, Lichtenberg (1989) places selfobject experiences of mirroring, idealization, and twinship within the attachment system. I am suggesting that the groupobject experiences are primarily aspects of affiliative motivations.

Summary

I have attempted to explore various aspects of the development of a theoretical perspective of group therapy as is evolved over the past 15 years. The evolution of this work has both anticipated and reflected the ongoing development of self psychology and advances in selfobject theory. Initially, the view of group events was primarily from a selfobject perspective, emphasizing the experiences of meeting or disrupting selfobject needs of individual group members. The focus was on healing empathic ruptures—a process that theoretically led to structure building. The addition of the multiple selfobject model suggested that the group setting makes possible selfobject experiences unavailable in individual treatment, thereby broadening and deepening access to the disturbances of the self. It was suggested that it was the opportunity for multiple selfobject experiences that made group therapy uniquely helpful in healing aspects of the self unavailable in individual therapy. This shift was soon followed by a series of enrichments based on the work of Stolorow et al. (1992), Lichtenberg et al. (1992), and Segalla (1995). In considering group from these additional perspectives, I find theoretical and clinical explanation for group processes that not only emphasizes the selfobject experiences of individual members, but also considers an array of clinical ideas that offer experience-near explanations for complex group events. These perspectives are particularly elegant for group treatment because they clear away many theoretical distractions and encourage work in the here and now, which is essential to group therapy. They also offer a model of group that acknowledges the relational experiences that are the bedrock of this form of treatment. While the model is based on theoretical advances from a dyadic treatment model, the ease of adaptation to a group speaks to the viability of the models explored. Selfobject theory, intersubjectivity, motivational systems, and groupobject theory all provide useful theoretical and clinical guides to the complex system of group therapy, and inform us about a given patient's self and their patterns of engagement with the other.

References

Bacal, H. (1985). Optimal responsiveness and the therapeutic process. In A. Goldberg (Ed.). *Progress in Self Psychology* (Vol. 1, pp. 202–227). New York: Guilford Press.

Beebe, B., & Lachmann, F. (1988). Mother–infant mutual influence and precursors of psychic structure. In A. Goldberg (Ed.), *Progress in self psychology*, (Vol. 3, pp. 3–25), Hillsdale, NJ: The Analytic Press.

Brandchaft, B. (1991). Countertransferance in the analytic process. *Progess in Self Psychology, 7*, 99–105.

Brandchaft, B. (1998). The self in developmental trauma. Paper presented at the 21st Annual Conference on the Psychology of the Self, San Diego, CA.

Galatzer-Levy, R. M., & Cohler, B. J. (1993). *The essential other: A developmental psychology of the self.* New York: Basic Books.

Harwood, I. (1986). The need for optimal available caretakers: Moving towards extended selfobject experience. *Group Analysis, 19*, 291–302.

Harwood, I. (1998). Advances in group psychotherapy and self psychology: An intersubjective approach. In I. Harwood & M. Pines (Eds.), *Self experiences in group: Intersubjective and self psychological pathways to human understanding* (pp. 30–47). London: Jessica Kingsley.

Kohut, H. (1959). Introspection, empathy and psychoanalysis. In P. Ornstein (Ed.), *The search for the self: selected writings of Heinz Kohut 1950–1978* (Vol. 1, pp. 205–232). New York: International Universities Press.

Kohut, H. (1976). Creativeness, charisma, group psychology. In P. Ornstein (Ed.), *The search for the self: Selected writings of Heinz Kohut, 1950–1978* (Vol. 2, pp. 793–843). New York: International Universities Press.

Kohut, H. (1984). In A. Goldberg & P. Stepansky (Eds.), *How does analysis cure?* Chicago: University of Chicago Press.

Lichtenberg, J. D. (1989). *Psychoanalysis and motivation.* Hillsdale, NJ: The Analytic Press.

Lichtenberg, J., Lachmann, F., & Fossage, J. (1992). *Self and motivational systems.* Hillsdale, NJ: The Analytic Press.

Paparo, F., & Nebbiosi, G. (1998). How does group cure? A reconceptualization of the group process: From self psychology to the intersubjective perspective. In I. Harwood & M. Pines (Eds.), *Self experiences in group: Intersubjective and self psychological pathways to human understanding* (pp. 70–83). London: Jessica Kingsley.

Segalla, R. A. (1985). Applications of self psychological principles to group psychotherapy. Unpublished paper. Presented to the Washington School of Psychiatry Philosophy of Psychotherapy Seminar, Washington, DC.

Segalla, R. A. (1995). The evolution of the self psychological perspective of group psychotherapy. Presented at the National Group Psychotherapy Training Institute, Washington, DC.

Segalla, R. A. (1996). "The unbearable embeddedness of being:" Self psychology, intersubjectivity and large group experiences. *Group, 20*, 4, 257–271.

Segalla, R. (1997). Recent advances in the application of self psychological principles to group psychotherapy. Presented at the 20th Annual Conference on the Psychoogy of Self, Chicago, IL.

Segalla, R., Silvers, D., Wine, B., & Pillsbury, S. (1988). Multiple selfobjects: Experiences in group and couples treatment. Presented at the 11th Annual Conference on the Psychology of the Self, Washington, DC.

Segalla, R., Silvers, D., Wine, B., & Pillsbury, S. (1988). Clinical applications of a multiple selfobject perspective in group and couples treatment. Presented at the 12th Annual Conference on the Psychology of the Self, San Francisco, CA.

Shapiro, E. (1998). Intersubjectivity in archaic and mature twinship in group therapy. In I. Harwood (Ed.), *Self experiences in group: Intersubjective and self psychological pathways to human understanding.* London and Philadelphia: Jessica Kingsley.

Silvers, D. L. (1998). A multiple selfobject and traumatizing experiences cotherapy model at work. In I. Harwood (Ed.), *Self experiences in group: Intersubjective and self psychological pathways to human understanding.* Jessica Kingsley.

Stolorow, R., & Atwood, G. (1992). *Contexts of being: The intersubjective foundations of psychological life.* Hillsdale, NJ: The Analytic Press.

Turquet, P. M. (1975). Threats to identity in the large group. In L. C. Kreeger (Ed.), *The large group dynamics and therapy* (pp. 87–144). London: Constable.

Wolf, K. (1988). *Treating the self.* New York: Guilford.

Toward Optimum Group Placement from the Perspective of the Self or Self-Experience

IRENE N. H. HARWOOD

This paper offers referring and prospective group analysts/therapists a way of conceptualizing optimum placement. This approach, using the charts provided, will aid in determining the patient's current needs based on past and present self-object functions, deficits/derailments, and traumatization. The charts also offer the group analyst/therapist a tool with which to evaluate the present selfobject functions, impingements, and traumatization that may be available in a prospective group to determine whether the match is appropriate or whether group should be the treatment modality of choice. When the interviewing analyst/therapist has taken all of the current and past selfobject functions and traumatization into account, the patient can be expected to benefit from the most growth-enhancing placement available.

Both Heinz Kohut (1977, 1984) and Donald Woods Winnicott (1965a, 1965b) saw development on a continuum. People with regressions or with derailed development along that continuum come to us with the hope of healing the pain or stagnation they are experiencing at whatever stage development was diverted.

Unless special care is given to patient selection and group composition, resumption of continued evolution along the potential developmental continuum will not occur. Worse yet, retraumatization and further regression can occur for the person with an already vulnerable self structure. Clinicians need a schema for patient selection to create an optimum group composition. The latter is a cornerstone of a working, healing group, which encompasses elements of "empathic selfobject ambiance" (Wolf, 1971/1980) and "optimal responsiveness" (Bacal & Newman, 1990). Without these elements the group environment can be less than optimum and the entire group can lose its potential healing power for an individual member.

Much has been written about the benefits of combining individual and group therapy (Harwood, 1983, 1986; Rutan & Stone, 1993; Segalla et al. 1989: Vinogradov & Yalom, 1989; Yalom, 1985) and, when that is impossible, of having preliminary individual sessions to obtain knowledge of genetic history) and to establish a firm selfobject bond between the group therapist and the potential group member (Harwood 1983, 1986).

The preliminary sessions are of extreme importance in determining optimum group placement: what kind of group is appropriate for what kind of person, whether one is selecting members for one's own groups, referring to another group therapist, or heading a group referral service.

This paper, through the use of charts based on theoretical concepts from the perspective of the self or self experience, will focus on the vulnerability and strengths of potential group members and will walk through what would constitute the most appropriate group placement. The relevance of early developmental deficits (Kohut, 1971, 1977, 1984), impingements (Winnicott, 1965a, 1965b), and traumas to current psychological structure as it relates to outside stressors will be explored. This understanding is necessary not only to evaluate an individual's functioning and developmental state in order to determine initial appropriate group placement, but also for the transferring of members from one type of group to another. It is important to recognize when a person may need to add, or move into, another type of group in order to provide different and currently more needed functions that would enable further growth on the developmental continuum.

Most individuals come to or are referred for treatment at a point of crisis or difficult transition in their lives. Their functioning may be regressed because of current external or internal impingements, which may or may not hark back to and join with earlier traumas. When present traumas join with earlier ones, they often become exponentially potentiated. The similarity of the traumas needs to be recognized as swiftly as possible. When the traumatic repetition is recognized and understood, the crisis begins to abate. What may look like psychosis can be understood not only as posttraumatic stress symptoms, but also as fragments of earlier traumatizations (often preverbal).

Therefore, looking at current functioning is not enough to understand what kind of treatment or group placement is needed. Knowledge of previous functioning, earlier deficits and impingements, and provisions of selfobject functions is critical for appropriate group placement. As group therapists/analysts know, an optimum group experience allows hope and transition to more optimum human relations in a person's life. A person can also experience currently and developmentally needed functions to restore a previous level of functioning.

In this paper I will share the manner in which I organize my thinking when I interview a patient. For this purpose I have developed several charts. The charts can be used to organize patient data systematically in order not to miss (1) the combining of earlier traumas with current ones and (2) either past or present needs for specific selfobject functions. I feel strongly that in order to understand a person's potentiality, one has to look at the present with an understanding of the past. Without both of these, one cannot understand the possible optimum, or retraumatizing, future.

First, I will explain the charts, which are shown at the end of the article, and then walk the reader through them with a potential group placement example.

By starting to follow Chart I, Selfobject Functions Available to Patients, we can determine what functions they had developmentally, which functions were good enough, which they did not have enough of, which they now have, which they lost, and which they never had. These functions are containing (Bion, 1952); soothing; protective (archaic idealized parental images, Kohut, 1971, 1977); structuralization of affects (differentiating, synthesizing, modulating, cognitively articulating, integrating affects, Socarides & Stolorow, 1984/1985); limit setting (Harwood, 1993); validation or mirroring of the total self (Kohut, 1977) or self-experience (Stolorow & Atwood, 1992); making room for idealization (Kohut, 1971, 1977); twinship experiences (Kohut, 1984); availability of fantasy/play (Bacal, 1992); multiple cross-cultural extended selfobject experiences (Harwood, 1986, 1993); allowance for self-delineation (Stolorow & Atwood, 1992); efficacy; and adversarial experiences (Wolf, 1971/1980).

Chart II helps us determine the Severity of Impingements and Traumas affecting a patient developmentally or currently and which are presently exponentially retraumatizing because of repetition and lack of the "protective function." These are internal impingements; external impingements; effectively disrupting continuity of being; physically derailing continuity of being; external interruption of creative gesture; substitution of creative gesture (Winnicott, 1965a, 1965b); physical molestation; sexual molestation; physical abuse; and sexual abuse.

Determining the overall picture on the first two charts gives us an overview of the developmental and current selfobject functions, environmental impingements, and traumas for Chart III, Patient Evaluation. In order to determine the cohesion and fragmentation (Kohut 1971, 1977) potential of the person's self-structure (not just looking at the current symptom or DSM-IV diagnosis), one needs to establish the current functioning level (as well as that person's previous highest functioning level). One cannot do this without determining, as much as possible, the levels of specific selfobject functions as well as the severity of internal and environmental impingements and traumas (developmentally and currently) assessed previously in Charts I and II.

To determine whether placement is appropriate in a psychoanalytic/psychodynamic group, rather than a supportive one, the person's capacities for tolerating disruptive affects, for self-boundary maintenance, for reestablishment of bonds, and for self-reflection must be determined. These, along with the absence of pronounced splitting, will help determine the degree of flexibility. Resilience can be assessed partly from previous capacity to restore functioning.

The assessment of a person's severity of deficits and traumatizations, as well as a person's flexibility and resilience, is extremely important in order to have some gauge for predicting affect tolerance (Socarides & Stolorow, 1984/1985) for working through within a therapeutic group, that is, the ability to deal with optimum frustrations (Kohut 1971, 1977), or withstand the breaking and reestablishing of selfobject bonds (Stolorow & Lachmann, 1984/1985). These factors are not only necessary for determining what the person needs (including who needs individual therapy and is not ready for group), but also if that person could be detrimental to others and should be excluded from group.

Chart IV is an Evaluation of Patients for Providing Potential Functions and Impingements/Traumatization for Others in a group. It is important to know this potential about everyone whom a group conductor is trying to bring together in a group: what functions they will provide for each other, how they might flare against each other, and how newcomers might affect individual members or the entire group. The potential functions are capacity for directness; capacity for mutuality/reciprocity (Kohut, 1977, 1984); and capacity for the use of empathy compassionately. The potential impingements or traumatizations are lack of self-restraint; failing to respect others' boundaries; and tendency to use empathy negatively or destructively (Kohut, 1981, 1984). Special attention should be paid to the potential to impinge or traumatize others. Patients prone to verbal or physically violent outbursts, who would violate confidentiality, or who would use the knowledge of someone's vulnerability to purposely hurt another should be excluded. One occurrence of the above should be heavily weighed before an exception is made to include that person in a heterogeneous group.

Table 1 presents an overview of different types of groups and which selfobject functions they might provide, thus helping in the selection of an optimal group for the patient. This table will help the clinician decide on the best type of group for the patient after determining the patient's current status and before going on to evaluate what potential functions and impingements a specific type of group-as-a-whole and its individual members can provide.

Chart V is an Evaluation of a Group and Individual Members for Providing Selfobject Functions needed by the patient. These are basically the same functions described in Chart I, but for the group. Chart VI is an Evaluation of a Group and Individual Members for Providing Potential Impingements, which would be too traumatizing for the patient at present. These are basically the same external impingements described in Chart II or possibly any other specific characteristics that a particular patient could not currently accept or tolerate.

CHART I
Selfobject Functions Available to Patients

SELFOBJECT FUNCTIONS	DEVELOPMENTALLY (-)....GOOD-ENOUGH....(+)	CURRENTLY (-)....GOOD-ENOUGH....(+)
A) CONTAINING		
B) SOOTHING		
C) PROTECTIVE		
D) STRUCTURALIZATION OF AFFECTS: Differentiating, Synthesizing, Modulating, Cognitively Articulating, and Integrating Affects		
E) LIMIT SETTING		
F) VALIDATION OR MIRRORING OF THE TOTAL SELF OR SELF/EXPERIENCE		
G) IDEALIZATION		
H) TWINSHIP/SAMENESS		
I) MULTIPLE CROSS-CULTURAL EXTENDED EXPERIENCES		
J) FANTASY/PLAY		
K) SELF-DELINEATION		
L) EFFICACY		
M) ADVERSARIAL EXPERIENCES		

CHART II
Severity of Impingements and Traumas

IMPINGEMENTS	DEVELOPMENTALLY (-)....GOOD-ENOUGH....(+)	CURRENTLY (-)....GOOD-ENOUGH....(+)
A) INTERNAL IMPINGEMENTS		
B) EXTERNAL IMPINGEMENTS		
C) AFFECTIVELY DISRUPTING CONTINUITY OF BEING		
D) PHYSICALLY DERAILING CONTINUITY OF BEING		
E) EXTERNAL INTERRUPTION OF CREATIVE GESTURES		
F) SUBSTITUTION OF CREATIVE GESTURES		
G) PHYSICAL MOLESTATION		
H) SEXUAL MOLESTATION		
I) PHYSICAL ABUSE		
J) SEXUAL ABUSE		

CHART III
Patient Evaluation

		(-)...............GOOD-ENOUGH................(+)		
SELFOBJECT FUNCTIONS AVAILABLE TO PATIENT (CHART I)	Developmentally			
	Currently			
SEVERITY OF IMPINGEMENTS AND TRAUMAS (CHART II)	Developmentally			
	Currently			
PATIENT'S				
CAPACITY FOR TOLERATING DISRUPTIVE AFFECTS				
CAPACITY FOR SELF-BOUNDARY MAINTENANCE				
CAPACITY FOR RE-ESTABLISHMENT OF BONDS				
CAPACITY FOR SELF-REFLECTION				
ABSENSE OF SPLITTING				
DEGREE OF FLEXIBILITY				
PREVIOUS CAPACITY TO RESTORE FUNCTIONING				
DEGREE OF RESILIENCE				
HIGHEST LEVEL OF FUNCTIONING	Previous			
	Current			
COHESION VS. FRAGMENTATION				

CHART IV
Evaluation of Patient for Providing Potential
Functions and Impingements/Traumatizations for Others

PATIENT'S	POTENTIAL FUNCTIONS (-) . . . . GOOD-ENOUGH . . . . (+)		
A) CAPACITY FOR DIRECTNESS			
B) CAPACITY FOR MUTUALITY/ RECIPROCITY			
C) CAPACITY FOR THE USE OF EMPATHY COMPASSIONATELY			
	POTENTIAL IMPINGEMENTS/TRAUMATIZATIONS		
D) LACK OF SELF-RESTRAINT			
E) FAILING TO RESPECT OTHERS' BOUNDARIES			
F) TENDENCY TO USE EMPATHY NEGATIVELY/ DESTRUCTIVELY			

TABLE 1
Selection of an Optimal Group

TYPES OF GROUPS:		A) CONTAINING	B) SOOTHING	C) PROTECTIVE	D) STRUCTURALIZATION OF AFFECTS	E) LIMIT SETTING	F) VALIDATION OR MIRRORING OF THE TOTAL SELF	G) IDEALIZATION	H) TWINSHIP/SAMENESS	I) MULTIPLE CROSS-CULTURAL EXTENDED EXPERIENCE	J) FANTASY/PLAY	K) SELF-DELINEATION	L) EFFICACY	M) ADVERSARIAL EXPERIENCES
ARCHAIC (A) MATURE (M) GOOD-ENOUGH (GE) NOT GOOD-ENOUGH (NGE)	SELFOBJECT FUNCTIONS:													
1) 12 STEP: OA AA GA														
2) EDUCATIONAL														
3) ADULT CHILDREN OF ALCOHOLICS (ACA)														
4) CODA														
5) ART THERAPY														
6) SYMPTOM SPECIFIC HOMOGENOUS: Divorce, Rape, Bulimia, & Support, etc.														
7) HETEROGENEOUS/ PSYCHODYNAMIC														
8) OBJECT RELATIONS														
9) SELF-PSYCHOLOGY														
10) INTEGRATED														

TABLE 1
Selection of an Optimal Group

TYPES OF GROUPS:	A) CONTAINING	B) SOOTHING	C) PROTECTIVE	D) STRUCTURALIZATION OF AFFECTS	E) LIMIT SETTING	F) VALIDATION OR MIRRORING OF THE TOTAL SELF	G) IDEALIZATION	H) TWINSHIP/SAMENESS	I) MULTIPLE CROSS-CULTURAL EXTENDED EXPERIENCE	J) FANTASY/PLAY	K) SELF-DELINEATION	L) EFFICACY	M) ADVERSARIAL EXPERIENCES
ARCHAIC (A)													
MATURE (M)													
GOOD-ENOUGH (GE)													
NOT GOOD-ENOUGH (NGE)													
1) 12 STEP: OA	A	GE	GE	0	✓	NGE	A	A	?	0	NGE	✓	0
AA	A	GE	GE	0	✓	NGE	A	A	?	0	NGE	✓	0
GA	A	GE	GE	0	✓	NGE	A	A	?	0	NGE	✓	0
2) EDUCATIONAL	✓	?	?	0	N/A	N/A	N/A	N/A	?	0	0	✓	0
3) ADULT CHILDREN OF ALCOHOLICS (ACA)	A	?	?	GE	A	?	?	A/M ?	?	0	NGE	✓	0
4) CODA	A	✓	✓	GE	A	?	A	A/M ?	?	0	NGE	✓	0
5) ART THERAPY	A/M ?	✓	N/A	?	N/A		?	M	?	M	?	✓	N/A
6) SYMPTOM SPECIFIC HOMOGENOUS: Divorce, Rape, Bulimia, & Support, etc.	✓	?	A	GE	N/A	part GE	GE?	A/M ?	?	0	GE	GE	0
7) HETEROGENEOUS/ PSYCHODYNAMIC	?	?	?	✓	?	✓	GE	M	?	?	✓	✓	✓
8) OBJECT RELATIONS Winnicott	?	?	?	✓	?	✓	GE	?	?	✓	✓	✓	?
Klein	?	?	?	✓	?	?	NGE eovy	?	?	?	✓	✓	✓
9) SELF-PSYCHOLOGY	✓	✓	✓	GE	GE	✓	M	M	?	?	✓	✓	GE
10) INTEGRATED	✓	✓	✓	GE	GE	✓	M	M	?	?	✓	✓	GE

SELFOBJECT FUNCTIONS:

CHART V
Evaluation of a Group and Individual Members
for Providing Selfobject Functions

SELFOBJECT FUNCTIONS	(-).................. GOOD-ENOUGH.................(+)		
A) CONTAINING			
B) SOOTHING			
C) PROTECTIVE			
D) STRUCTURALIZATION OF AFFECTS: Differentiating, Synthesizing, Modulating, Cognitively Articulating, and Integrating Affects			
E) LIMIT SETTING			
F) VALIDATION OR MIRRORING OF THE TOTAL SELF OR SELF/EXPERIENCE			
G) IDEALIZATION			
H) TWINSHIP/SAMENESS			
I) MULTIPLE CROSS-CULTURAL EXTENDED EXPERIENCES			
J) FANTASY/PLAY			
K) SELF-DELINEATION			
L) EFFICACY			
M) ADVERSARIAL EXPERIENCES			

CHART VI
Evaluation of a Group and Individual Members
for Providing Potential Impingements

(CHART I) POTENTIAL IMPINGEMENTS	(-)...................GOOD-ENOUGH.....................(+)		
C) AFFECTIVELY DISRUPTING CONTINUITY OF BEING			
D) PHYSICALLY DERAILING CONTINUITY OF BEING			
E) EXTERNAL INTERRUPTION OF CREATIVE GESTURES			
F) SUBSTITUTION OF CREATIVE GESTURES			
G) OTHER SPECIFIC INTOLERABLE CHARACTERISTICS			

Case Illustration

The reader will now be introduced to "Abigail." The details that Abigail presented in her initial interview are summarized. The data will be used to walk the evaluating clinician through the use of the charts.

Abigail has recently been raped. She is 29, Caucasian, single, and had been in an abusive heterosexual relationship. Her boyfriend blamed her for the rape and was not sensitive to her terror or flashbacks. She felt angry and abandoned by him and they stopped seeing each other.

She feels somewhat responsible for causing the rape by somehow not preventing the intruder from forcing entry into her house. Following up on these feelings of responsibility, she reveals sexual molestation by a paternal uncle. Also, she relates, her own father had often made inappropriate sexual comments about how she looked. When she looked toward her mother, her mother looked away.

Abigail feels her mother loves her since her mother always shares her problems with Abigail, including feeling somewhat abused by her current husband. Abigail feels she is stronger than her mother since her younger brother and sister come to her for advice and protection. There are vague memories of being cared for and loved by a maternal grandmother who died when she was 5 years old.

Abigail is exhibiting posttraumatic stress disorder symptoms. Though she has always been successfully employed in a creative profession, she is having trouble concentrating or considering herself a worthwhile employee. She is demeaning herself after being demeaned by the violation. The current violation is potentiated by the molestations, impingements, and lack of protection against these in her past. She is still frightened around men, but appears more trusting of women. Recently, three of her closest women friends moved away. Her female employer has validated her work in the past and appears to be understanding of her recent posttraumatic situation. Abigail is afraid that this understanding will run out if her concentration, productivity, and creativity do not soon return to her previous level of functioning.

From what Abigail described about her recent long-distance phone conversations with the friends who moved, she is able to benefit from their empathy and support and able to ask about, listen to, and comment on their concerns. But she is often left longing for more because she cannot have them close by and ends up crying and remembering her long-gone grandmother. She refrains from calling them daily, for fear both of using up their availability and of running up excessive phone bills, since she has retained a lawyer to help her prosecute the rapist "in order not to feel like a total victim."

Chart I reveals what kind of caring functions have been available to Abigail in the past and in the present. It appears that both mother and, particularly, grandmother have validated her and the unique qualities that have helped Abigail develop and pursue her talents and creativity. The grandmother has also extended some protective, assertive functions, which allow Abigail to reach out for help to female friends, to a therapist, and to an attorney. With additional protective, containing, and encouraging functions for her to articulate her rage, rather than containing alone her disintegrating affects, she will most likely be able to integrate them assertively and efficaciously, if they are provided in a therapeutic situation. A tendency for her to join with the affects of others, such as has been the case with her mother, would need to be watched to prevent her from getting sidetracked from delineating her own feelings and needs from those of others.

In looking at Abigail's impingements and traumas on Chart II, we see that her past as well as her more recent relations with men have been of an abusive and traumatizing nature. If she feels she can tolerate being with men and speaking about her situation in a group, the men in the potential group should have the ability to be understanding and empathic and have sustained some breakthrough of their own physical/psychological boundaries. If she cannot at present be in the presence of men, if the aura of the abuser has been generalized to most males, she should either be seen individually by a female therapist or be in an all-female group (not necessarily a symptom-specific one). Eventually, though, transition into a group with empathic males would be essential in order for her not to repeat her choices and conflicts in her early male relations. A consistent availability of caring, respectful, reciprocal functions from male group members could help her both heal the early and recent traumas and look toward more equal and respectful relationships with males.

Chart III shows that although Abigail's current cohesion and functioning are less than optimum, it is clear from her multitude of capacities that she has been at a much higher level most of her life and could probably return to that level if safeguarded from other impingements and traumas and provided with needed, healing functions.

Considering Abigail's direct and appropriate manner in the interview, as well as her reports that she is able to be giving to her now long-distance friends, she would be a positive contributor in almost any group, as is shown on Chart IV. It is not clear at this point how she would interact in a group where male (or female) members would be dominating or impinging in some way. She definitely would need to be safeguarded from being retraumatized; therefore, groups with high levels of confrontation, conflict, or verbal aggression should be avoided.

Table 1 gives a quick overview of how the structure of specific types of groups would (√) or would not (0) provide certain functions, particularly those that Abigail would especially require. Except for those groups with a particular agenda or structure, the functions or impingements that a particular group may provide will largely depend on the style and theoretical orientation of the group conductor, after which groups tend to model themselves. Otherwise, the healing or traumatizing potential of a group will depend on the qualities of the individual members, on the balance and diversity of the group composition, and on what an individual group member experiences as "optimally frustrating" (Kohut, 1971, 1977) or affectively tolerable.

Charts V and VI evaluate a specific group and group members for the potential functions and impingements they might provide for Abigail. The males have either had similar impingements or can be positively present or empathic to Abigail. Only one female possesses some selfish, abrasive qualities, which, because of the same sex component, would probably not be transferentially too traumatizing for Abigail, but instead, with modeling by the rest of the group, allow Abigail to practice her needed self-delineation, adversarial, and efficacy functions.

CHART I
Selfobject Functions Available to Patients
(Example: Abigail)

SELFOBJECT FUNCTIONS		DEVELOPMENTALLY		CURRENTLY
A)	CONTAINING		grandmother appeared to have served these functions	no one to talk to since female friends moved away
B)	SOOTHING			
C)	PROTECTIVE		(? grandmother) since A. able to protect siblings	stayed in abusive, blaming relationship
D)	STRUCTURALIZATION OF AFFECTS: Differentiating, Synthesizing, Modulating, Cognitively Articulating, and Integrating Affects	mother did not likely differentiate A.'s affects from her own	? not clear what grandmother did	mother uses her for discharging her own affects
E)	LIMIT SETTING		?	she needs to set limits with mother
F)	VALIDATION OR MIRRORING OF THE TOTAL SELF OR SELF/EXPERIENCE	father verbally abusive of her physical self	mother validated her creativity not total self	appears there is no one currently
G)	IDEALIZATION		grandmother	woman boss
H)	TWINSHIP/SAMENESS	sees herself as victim like her mother		mother still archaically merged
I)	MULTIPLE CROSS-CULTURAL EXTENDED EXPERIENCES		?	2 best friends were of different culture
J)	FANTASY/PLAY		apparently allowed because of creativity	in her work only
K)	SELF-DELINEATION		not clear if allowed earlier	mother requires merger
L)	EFFICACY			was able to be creative & productive at work
M)	ADVERSARIAL EXPERIENCES			(-) not able to escape rape (+) retaining attorney

CHART II
Severity of Impingements and Traumas
(Example: Abigail)

IMPINGEMENTS	DEVELOPMENTALLY (-)....GOOD-ENOUGH.....(+)	CURRENTLY (-)....GOOD-ENOUGH.....(+)
A) INTERNAL IMPINGEMENTS	?	SHAME
B) EXTERNAL IMPINGEMENTS	1) abuse by uncle 2) inappropiate behavior by father 3) maternal affects	(-) ! current rape
C) AFFECTIVELY DISRUPTING CONTINUITY OF BEING	mother requires A. to feel like her	recent boyfriend's blaming and berating
D) PHYSICALLY DERAILING CONTINUITY OF BEING	uncle father	flashback of rape
E) EXTERNAL INTERRUPTION OF CREATIVE GESTURES	✓	
F) SUBSTITUTION OF CREATIVE GESTURE	✓	(+) good woman boss
G) PHYSICAL MOLESTATION	father	
H) SEXUAL MOLESTATION	uncle	
I) PHYSICAL ABUSE		
J) SEXUAL ABUSE	uncle	(-) rape

CHART III
Patient Evaluation
(Example: Abigail)

(-) . . . . GOOD-ENOUGH . . . .(+)

A) SELFOBJECT FUNCTIONS AVAILABLE TO PATIENT (CHART I)	Developmentally		mother did not protect	mother validated creativity	grandmother
	Currently	3 friends moved away	mother merges, burdens with own problems		woman employer validating and understanding
B) SEVERITY OF IMPINGEMENTS AND TRAUMAS (CHART II)	Developmentally	1) molestation by uncle 2) verbal, sexualized abuse by father			
	Currently	1) RAPE 2) recent abusive relationship	mother impinges with own affect		
PATIENT'S					
C) CAPACITY FOR TOLERATING DISRUPTIVE AFFECTS				able to hang onto self regardless of mother	
D) CAPACITY FOR SELF-BOUNDARY MAINTENANCE				✓	
E) CAPACITY FOR RE-ESTABLISHMENT OF BONDS				✓	
F) CAPACITY FOR SELF-REFLECTION				✓	
G) ABSENCE OF SPLITTING				? not evident	
H) DEGREE OF FLEXIBILITY					✓
I) PREVIOUS CAPACITY TO RESTORE FUNCTIONING				✓	
J) DEGREE OF RESILIENCE				✓	
K) HIGHEST LEVEL OF FUNCTIONING	Previous				✓
	Current		✓	at present regression	
L) COHESION VS. FRAGMENTATION			✓	future potential	

CHART IV
Evaluation of Patient for Providing Potential
Functions and Impingements/Traumatizations for Others
(Example: Abigail)

PATIENT'S	POTENTIAL FUNCTIONS (-) . . . . GOOD-ENOUGH . . . . (+)		
A) CAPACITY FOR DIRECTNESS			√
B) CAPACITY FOR MUTUALITY/ RECIPROCITY			with friends even when she is needy
C) CAPACITY FOR THE USE OF EMPATHY COMPASSIONATELY			√
	POTENTIAL IMPINGEMENTS/TRAUMATIZATIONS		
D) LACK OF SELF-RESTRAINT		no indication	
E) FAILING TO RESPECT OTHERS' BOUNDARIES		no indication	
F) TENDENCY TO USE EMPATHY NEGATIVELY/ DESTRUCTIVELY		no indication	

TABLE 1
Selection of an Optimal Group
(Example: Abigail)

TYPES OF GROUPS: SELFOBJECT FUNCTIONS:

ARCHAIC (A)
MATURE (M)
GOOD-ENOUGH (GE)
NOT GOOD-ENOUGH (NGE)

TYPES OF GROUPS	A) CONTAINING	B) SOOTHING	C) PROTECTIVE	D) STRUCTURALIZATION OF AFFECTS	E) LIMIT SETTING	F) VALIDATION OR MIRRORING OF THE TOTAL SELF	G) IDEALIZATION	H) TWINSHIP/SAMENESS	I) MULTIPLE CROSS-CULTURAL EXTENDED EXPERIENCE	J) FANTASY/PLAY	K) SELF-DELINEATION	L) EFFICACY
1) 12 STEP: OA AA GA	not applicable											
2) EDUCATIONAL	not applicable											
3) ADULT CHILDREN OF ALCOHOLICS (ACA)	not applicable											
4) CODA	not applicable											
5) ART THERAPY ?	√	maybe	N/A	only if content of art articulated	N/A	?	?	0	?	√	?	?
6) SYMPTOM SPECIFIC HOMOGENOUS: Divorce, Rape, Bulimia, & Support, etc.	√	?	A	only if articulating the affects experienced after the rape	N/A	GE	GE?	A	?	NGE	GE	GE
7) HETEROGENEOUS/ PSYCHODYNAMIC	depends on group conductor and composition											
8) OBJECT RELATIONS	depends if Winnicottian / Kleinian / Kernbergian & group conductors											
9) SELF-PSYCHOLOGY	depends on group conductor and composition											
10) INTEGRATED	depends on group conductor and composition											

CHART V
Evaluation of a Group and Individual Members
for Providing Selfobject Functions
(Example: Abigail)

SELFOBJECT FUNCTIONS	(-)...............	GOOD-ENOUGH..............	(+)
A) CONTAINING			no difficulty with strong affect
B) SOOTHING	one female abrasive in manner		soflty spoken except for one
C) PROTECTIVE			males culturally protective of females
D) STRUCTURALIZATION OF AFFECTS: Differentiating, Synthesizing, Modulating, Cognitively Articulating, and Integrating Affects			very articulate intelligent differentiating of affects group
E) LIMIT SETTING		potential practicing with abrasive female member	
F) VALIDATION OR MIRRORING OF THE TOTAL SELF OR SELF/EXPERIENCE	one mother puts emphasis on physical attractiveness of partners (only)	√	
G) IDEALIZATION		intelligent articulate caring group	
H) TWINSHIP/SAMENESS		male member molested by brother	
I) MULTIPLE CROSS-CULTURAL EXTENDED EXPERIENCES			homosexual heterosexual different religions three different ethnicities/races
J) FANTASY/PLAY		humor and use of metaphor	
K) SELF-DELINEATION		ask what each feels or wants	
L) EFFICACY		encouragement achievement assertiveness	
M) ADVERSARIAL EXPERIENCES		potential practicing with abrasive female member	

CHART VI
Evaluation of a Group and Individual Members
for Providing Potential Impingements
(Example: Abigail)

(CHART I) POTENTIAL IMPINGEMENTS	(-)............... GOOD-ENOUGH ....(+)		
C) AFFECTIVELY DISRUPTING CONTINUITY OF BEING		only one member interrupts, at times inappropriately when in narcissistic need	
D) PHYSICALLY DERAILING CONTINUITY OF BEING			none
E) EXTERNAL INTERRUPTION OF CREATIVE GESTURES			none (creative gestures are recognized or applauded
F) SUBSTITUTION OF CREATIVE GESTURES	any different ideas & solutions which could be difficult for fragmented self		
G) OTHER SPECIFIC INTOLERABLE CHARACTERISTICS		none	

Conclusions

Abigail's charting after her first evaluation interview indicates that she is ready for treatment. Before going further, however, it should first be established whether Abigail—or any potential group member—is ready for an analytic heterogeneous group. If she is, further interviews with the prospective group therapist should be held to gather historical information that will be helpful for interventions when transferential material with other members emerges, and for the establishment of a firm selfobject bond that the patient can rely on when the transferential material with other group members becomes too conflictual and threatens retraumatization.

On one hand, if a mixed-sex group is found to be too threatening for the potential group member, the interviewing therapist should determine if the patient needs, wants, and has established enough of a connection to the interviewing therapist to continue in individual sessions before considering any other type of group. It should always be left in the control of the patient to make the final decision. This is particularly crucial for patients who have been severely impinged, traumatized, and controlled in any portion of their lives.

At the end of the interview, patients should be asked if they feel comfortable enough to continue working with the same clinician. If the connection with the interviewing therapist/analyst is determined to be "not good-enough" (Winnicott, 1965a), patients should be referred elsewhere.

On the other hand, if the connection is "good-enough," but the potential group member is too fearful to be in a mixed-sex group at this time, or is in great need of an archaic twinship experience (to know that others have gone through a similar experience and have similar feelings), and if the interviewing therapist does not have a same-issue, single-sex group, referral to a same-symptom group (which can also function as an educational group) may be the first step to a very normalizing, healing, and supportive experience.

The same-symptom group should never be a total substitute for a heterogeneous analytical group. A heterogeneous group is a necessary step for readying oneself to deal with different aspects of the world, including sorting out and working through transferential aspects that otherwise could be experienced as retraumatizing. A heterogeneous group also provides many diverse cross-cultural extended experiences (Harwood, 1986, 1993), which offer many unknown and unconsidered windows of possibility, discoveries, and growth in a person's life.

Unfortunately, the simplistic formulas and the narrow-minded requirements of managed care, insurance companies, and the evolving health care systems of many countries are placing individuals needing developmental growth into symptom or behavior ghettoes that in the long run may be no better than racial/ethnic/religious/socioeconomic ghettoes. Eventually, this type of compartmentalization can restrict patients' awareness of the diversity and universality of human feelings. Learning that those different from our selves, but who possess the important capacity for empathy, can understand us and reach out to us simply as one ordinary human being to another can in a profound human experience. Such a group experience reaches outside of the group therapy culture and further enhances human fellowship among other diverse groups. It can contribute to global understanding and concern for people who look and appear different from ourselves.

Feeling understood by people like ourselves is structure enhancing. Feeling that no one who is unlike ourselves (with different experiences or characteristics) can understand us closes the door on any trust or hope about the universality of human feelings or human empathy. Only when we have been understood and respected by others unlike ourselves can we walk with some modicum of trust and safety in the universe.

In Abigail's case, she went on to make a "good-enough" selfobject bond with the interviewing therapist to complete six preliminary sessions. With some trepidation, she joined the heterogeneous group that the interviewing therapist conducted. (If the interviewing therapist did not have such a group, inquiring about aspects of other appropriate groups available would have been the next step.)

Not long after Abigail joined the group, she thought she saw her rapist on the street. She felt she could not return to the group because one of the men in the group seemed to have physical characteristics similar to the rapist. (The characteristics of the perpetrator were starting to spread globally.) She returned for individual sessions with the group conductor to work on the post traumatic stress disorder symptoms. After a couple of sessions, she was able to return to group, because of the already established strong selfobject tie with the therapist in the preliminary sessions, and was able to bring up and work through the transferential aspects with the support and compassion of the male members in particular.

By utilizing the specific information gleaned from the charts, Abigail was placed in a group where she was able to heal and to continue to grow. Ever after seeing the rapist at the beginning of her group experience caused a disruption in the selfobject bond with the group, she was able to utilize the established selfobject bond with the group conductor to return to the group and to allow the empathic understanding of the group members to help reestablish the bond with the entire group, thereby moving toward further integrating the difference between the male members of this group and past perpetrators in her life.

Through the use of these charts the group conductor can gain very detailed and specific understanding of the potential selfobject functions, impingements, and self-delineation and empathic capacities of the group members. This specific understanding helps to address more subtlety the past strengths and potential growth of the patient, thus to fine tune an optimum growth placement.

Patients who possess the capacities to endure the disruptions and reconnections of a psychoanalytic/psychodynamic group should not be held back by a group that does not allow their potential to stretch. A group that is run from a focus on the perspective of self, or self-experience, allows for the healing process of the disruption and reconnection sequences of selfobject bonds to take place. Beebe, Jaffe, and Lachman's (1992) research confirms that it is not the perfect merger between mother and child that builds psychic structure, but the number of disconnection-reconnection sequences between them.

Group analysts/therapists can continue to evolve in their healing and build-ing of further psychic structure of their patients, not through maintaining archaic merger or archaic twinship, but by developmentally moving each individual group member toward more mature selfobject functioning and resolution of conflicts, as well as toward mutuality and reciprocity. Hopefully, the system of charts pre-sented in this paper will contribute to this process.

References

Bacal, H. (1992). *Selfobject relationships redefined*. Paper presented at the Self Psychol-ogy Conference, Los Angeles.

Bacal, H., & Newman, K. (1990). *Theories of object relations: bridges to self psychology*. New York: Columbia University Press.

Beebe, B., Jaffe, J., & Lachman, F. (1992). A dyadic systems view of communication. In N. Skolnick & S. Warshaw (Eds.), *Relational perspectives in psychoanalysis*. Hill-sdale, NJ: Analytic Press.

Bion, W. R. (1952). Group dynamics: A review. *International Journal of Psychoanalysis, 33*, 235–247.

Harwood, I. (1983). The application of self psychology to group psychotherapy. *Interna-tional Journal of Group Psychotherapy, 33*, 469–487.

Harwood, I. (1986). The need for optimal, available caretakers: Moving towards extended selfobject experience. *Group Analysis, 19*, 291–302.

Harwood, T. (1993). *Examining early childhood multiple cross-cultural extended self-object and traumatic experiences and creating optimum treatment environments*. Paper presented at the Self Psychology Conference, Toronto.

Kohut. H. (1971). *The analysis of the self*. New York: International Universities Press.

Kohut, H. (1977). *The restoration of the self*. New York International Universities Press.

Kohut, H. (1984). *How does analysis cure?* Chicago: University of Chicago Press.

Rutan, J. S., & Stone, W. N. (1993). *Psychodynamic group psychotherapy* (2nd ed.). New York: Guilford Press.

Segalla, R., Silvers, D., Wine, B., & Pillsbury, G. (1989). *Multiple selfobject relationships*. Paper presented at the Self Psychology Conference, San Francisco.

Socarides, D. D., & Stolorow, R. D. (1984/1985). Affects and selfobjects. *Annual of Psy-choanalysis, 12*(13),105–119.

Stolorow, R. D., & Atwood, G. E. (1992). *Contexts of being*. Hillsdale, NJ: Analytic Press.

Stolorow, R. D., & Lachmann, F. M. (1984/1985). Transference: The future of an illusion. *Annual of Psychoanalysis, 12*(13), 19–37.

Vinogradov, S., & Yalom, I. (1989). *A concise guide to group psychotherapy*. Washington, DC: American Psychiatric Press.

Winnicott, D. W. (1965a). Ego distortion in terms of the true and false self. In *The matu-rational processes and the facilitating environment*. New York: International Uni-versities Press.

Winnicott, D. W. (1965b). The theory of the parent-infant relationship. In *The matura-tional processes and the facilitating environment*. New York: International Univer-sities Press.

Wolf, E. A. (1980). On the developmental line of selfobject relations. In A. Goldberg (Ed.), *Advances in self psychology*. London: Tavistock Publications. (Original work published 1971)

Yalom, I. (1985). *The theory and practice of group psychotherapy*. New York: Basic Books.

Anger in Group Therapy
A Self Psychological Perspective

MARY DLUHY

Self Psychology as a psychoanalytic theory beginning with Heinz Kohut in the 1970s is now in its third decade. As the theory has evolved, the way self psychology looks at aggression and anger has been a controversial matter.

Self psychology is not focused on drive-related instinctual conflict or motives, but is examining the internal experience of deficits where hurt and injury predominate. With empathy being the cornerstone of the theory, many people in psychoanalytic circles have believed that self psychologists disregard anger and aggression or attempt to soothe them away. Empathy as defined by Kohut does not mean collusion or agreement, rather it is a form of intervention and central in the development of the therapeutic relationship. It refers to the method by which the therapist comes to understand the patient's internal experience.

From a self psychological perspective, before anger or aggression is analyzed, injury, hurt or damage to self-worth is examined. For some patients, a deeper danger is the lack of any self-assertion, where assertion or anger is split off into a depleted self; this is a state of little or no self worth. At the other end of this spectrum are those with unlimited grandiosity, the defense against a depleted self-worth, two sides to the same coin.

Psychoanalysis has long recognized aggression as a central motivator of human actions. On a continuum, aggression is agency to get up and go as well as courage to take on new challenges. It can also be healthy entitlement, which might include assertion, disappointment, frustration, or adversity. On the other hand, depending on internal structure, it may be a destructive force that without successful sublimation can be violent (Alonso, 1995).

In self psychology, aggression is seen as inborn, while anger is object connected or a break in the selfobject transference. Heinz Kohut distinguished two types of aggression, those being competitive aggression, directed at objects that stand in the way of goals and ambitions, and narcissistic rage, directed at selfobjects who threaten or have actually damaged the self (Wolf, 1988). These two types of aggression are structurally different and have very different psychological consequences.

Competitive aggressiveness is the normal, healthy reaction to obstacles that hinder the attainment of the individual's aims in the world. It is the energy with which we build and change our environment; it disappears or lessens when the hurdle that evoked it is overcome. Some of us have more of this aggression than others, which depends on many factors, including character, genes, and our surround.

Narcissistic rage, the other form of aggression described by Kohut, is a more complex issue. The origin of this rage is in response to the state of helplessness, shame, or emptiness vis-à-vis the humiliating, idealized selfobject caregiver which may have been too intrusive, too provocative or a lack of response, that is, a nonmirroring environment or injuries to grandiosity.

Such experiences are unbearably painful as they threaten the very continuity and existence of the self. The rage is coming from a self that is desperately attempting to reconstitute or maintain its identity. Narcissistic rage does not vanish when the offense is over. The painful memory lingers on, as does the resentment. At some point, the smoldering animosity is likely to break out in revenge, open hostility, or perhaps cold, calculating destructiveness. It finds its satisfaction in victimizing a stand-in selfobject who has offended. Narcissistic rage is seen in those with identity or selfobject impairment where there has been a failure in the phase-appropriate response from the selfobject caregivers (Stone, 1995). Interpretation has very little effect in these episodes and, in fact, can be more injurious or seen as criticism or blame. As Howard Bacal has aptly stated, one cannot apply unmodified classical drive theory in this clinical situation and expect that the patient will feel understood.

In group therapy, after a rageful explosion, other group members may feel angry or frightened, which can cause alienation and perhaps paranoia. This is a place for self psychology to intervene, not to protect, but to get inside the cycle. What is being experienced in the process? This is a tricky spot, where the rageful individual can get scapegoated by the group or may threaten to leave the group. The therapist's narcissism may get tapped into at this point as well. He or she might get angry at the patient for disrupting the group, or at the patient's help rejecting attitude. At a deeper level, the patient may strike at the therapist's sadism or masochism.

A group-as-a-whole intervention may take some of the pressure off this individual. For example, "I wonder what x is holding for all of us, or why has this come up now?" This is an attempt to hold and detoxify these unbearable feelings, and get the group working on an intersubjective understanding of what this individual is trying to regulate in him or herself and in the group. The group-as-a-whole intervention also reminds that there are no innocent bystanders (Gans, 1989). If the group can tolerate the regression, this will build the group ego, a groupobject need (Segalla, 1998). We also must remind ourselves that there are times when any and all interventions fail.

A clinical vignette illustrates this. Betty was a member of a long-term weekly group. For a long period of time, with many repetitions, if someone in the group said something Betty believed was emotionally dishonest, she would begin to attack the individual in an angry, belligerent way. Often, depending on the person and circumstances, for example, the group colluding with the individual's feelings or position, Betty would become rageful. If I intervened in any way to check out what was going on, or if I didn't intervene, she attacked me for side taking or for being passive, impotent and generally, "not getting what's going on." At these times, the group was clearly unsafe for her, and she would threaten to leave the group. She was also falling into the group scapegoat position, where she is the "group problem."

These episodes in the group repeated family of origin material. Betty was raised in a poor, Catholic Irish family with six siblings. In her view, her father was overly dominating, aggressive, and narcissistic, while mother was passive, depressed, and ineffective at problem solving. Betty was the one who cried foul when things in the family felt "crazy" to her. When she did this, family members turned on her. She became the "family problem."

In the group, her internal experience in the family was getting repeated. Interpreting the family of origin material, where I was "acting" like the passive, incompetent mother and the other group members were ganging up on her like her siblings, or any variation of what this felt like for her in the group, made matters worse. It heightened her paranoia and left her feeling that she was and is alone. Time and time again, this remained unfinished business in the group with little or not metabolizing any of the parts. Betty was far too injured and vulnerable to see she was taking on the role of her father in the group by becoming belligerent and attacking.

Self psychology supports the combined use of group and individual treatment. The combination provides the "multiple selfobject field" (Segalla et al., 1987), which may hold the most promise for deep disturbance. It was in the individual treatment, where Betty was less exposed, where we could begin to explore what her experience was like just before one of those rages in the group. This was deep, painful, and difficult to access and was at the actual level of self deficit. It was the utter helplessness, shame, and humiliation she experienced as a child with her angry father and helpless mother. She felt alone, terrified and anxious; deep, timorous, disintegrating anxiety. When she and I could get through this with my taking in her alienation and fear, by experiencing my own impotence and helplessness, and bit by bit by tolerating and holding these feelings and describing them to her, she began to internalize a strengthened self. Internal structure was changing, narcissism was moving upwards from a primitive grandiosity (Ashbach, 1995). She was finally able to hold and put words on her fears and anxiety and begin to experience that she wasn't "crazy." Yvonne Agazarian writes that the containment of hatred without a target is the nexus of the healing experience (Agazarian, 1994).

As Betty took this back into the group, she asked the group for help in announcing or describing her feelings and checking in on herself when the feelings of needing to attack arose. With a strengthened self, she was able to go into the exploration of her affects as signals and found ways to express the fears without rage.

Important here is to make the distinction between narcissistic injury or rupture and narcissistic rage. They are points on the continuum of object relatedness. As Jerry Gans says in his article, "Hostility in Group Psychotherapy," one of the most frequent forms of hostility in groups is narcissistic injury. Injury or slight can be held by the individual, and often the anger or hurt is expressed. Narcissistic rage is explosive and rejecting of the inter-personal bond. It is as if there were no history or object constancy of self or other. Simply put, injury is alienation, versus annihilation in rage. In injury, self-esteem is wounded, but it is not injurious at the core. It is a hurt or a slight at someone else's hands, and is most often grist for the therapeutic mill. Injuries happen frequently in group and, although painful, are how ruptures are understood and worked through (Gans, 1989). Betty fell somewhere between these two on the continuum. Narcissistic injuries are problematic and serious only if the patient, group, or leader does not ascertain the injury and the patient leaves the group, painfully repeating old damage.

Self psychology is a relatively new theory and, consistent with development, there are many other milestones to achieve in integrating an understanding the complex area of self-assertion, aggression, and anger. As the theory has progressed new conceptualization of assertion, adversity and aggression have emerged as well.

In 1988, Ernest Wolf added efficacy and adversarial to the selfobject needs along with mirroring, idealizing and alter-ego.

In Lichtenberg, Lachman and Fosshage's *Self and Motivational Systems,* two of the five motivational systems describe aggression: (3) the need for exploration an assertion and (4) the need to react aversively through antagonism or withdrawal (or both).

From an intersubjective perspective as advanced by Stolorow and Atwood all affect states including ruptures, anger, and rage must be understood within the context of the experience both past and present. Intersubjectivity as a system of reciprocal influence has taken us much farther along in our understanding of the rupture/repair sequence of treatment.

Conclusion

To summarize, self psychology is attempting to get underneath the deficit to the deeper internal experience. This is achieved through mirroring, empathetic introspection, and the use of the intersubjective experience. In our more damaged patients, hurt, injury, and deep pain are often what predominate through the earlier phases of treatment. We are working with damaged self-worth, a depleted self, where we do not see anger per se, rather aggression turned inward, against the self. This takes many forms, for example, depression or unrelenting masochism from which it is felt there is no exit. The patient who comes with grandiosity and entitlement may lead with aggression in the form of an overdose of competitive aggression or narcissistic rage, but again, these are defenses against a depleted self. Generally, assertion, anger, and aggression come through the treatment as the self-worth is strengthened.

References

Ashbach, C., & Schermer, V. (1992). In *Handbook of Contemporary Group Psychotherapy*, R. Klein, H. Bernard, D. Singer. Madison CT: International Universities Press, pp. 219–319.

Alonso, A. (1995). Discussant comments for special section on anger and aggression in groups. *International Journal of Group Psychotherapy*, *45*, pp. 331–338.

Agazarian. Y. (1994). The phrases of group development and the systems centered group. In *Ring of Fire*, ed. V. Schermer & M. Pines. London: Routledge, pp. 36–838.

Bacal, H. (1992). Contributions from self psychology theory. In, *Handbook of Contemporary Group Psychotherapy*, ed. R. Klein, H. Bernard, D. Singer. Madison, CT: International Universities Press. pp. 55–83.

Gans, J. (1989). Hostility in group psychotherapy. *International Journal of Group Psychotherapy*, *39*, 499–516.

Harwood, I. (1992). Advances in group psychotherapy and self psychology: An intersubjective approach. *Group*, *16*, 4, Winter 1992, pp. 220–232.

Lichtenberg, J. D., Lachman, F. M., & Fosshage, J. L. (1992). *Self and Motivational System Toward a Theory of Psychoanalytic Technique*. Hillsdale, NJ. The Analytic Press.

Segalla, R. Silvers, D. & Wine, B. (1987). Paper presentations on Groups' Multiple Selfobject. National Self Psychology Conference.

Segalla, R. (1998). Motivational systems and groupobject theory: Implications for group therapy. In: *Self Experience in Group: Intersubjective and Self Psychological Pathways to Human Understanding*, ed. I. N. H. Harwood and M. Pines. London, England: Jessica Kingsley Publishers, LTD, pp. 141–155.

Stolorow, R., & Atwood, G. (1992). *Context of Being: The Intersubjective Foundations of Psychological Life*. Hillsdale, NJ: The Analytic Press.

Stone, W. (1995). Frustration, anger, and the significance of alter-ego transferences in group psychotherapy. *International Journal of Group Psychotherapy*, *45*, pp. 287–302.

Wolf, E. S. (1988). *Treating the Self Elements of Clinical Self Psychology*. New York: The Guilford Press.

Working With Intersubjectivity

Mary Dluhy

One of self psychology's main contributions to psychoanalytic theory is that it has provided new ways of conceptualizing the therapeutic process. It has aided us in our continuing understanding of how treatment "works" or what actually happens in therapy.

Heinz Kohut's conceptualization of transmuting internalization as the under-standing/explaining sequence of ruptures in treatment brought us a clearer view of childhood's unmet needs and deficits in the development. These are reacti-vated in the therapeutic situation, through what Kohut called optimal frustration (Kohut, 1984). This is when the therapist inevitably fails the patient, the patient is injured in a reactivation of an old wound, and an opportunity presents itself to begin repair of some early damage.

As time has gone on, there has been some evolution in the concept of optimal frustration to optimal responsiveness. This term coined by Howard Bacal in the book *Theories of Object Relations: Bridges to Self Psychology* includes both the patient's experience of frustration and the therapist's response to needs; Bacal moved us closer to viewing the therapist's role in interventions. While empa-thy refers to the method by which the therapist comes to understand the patient, optimal responsiveness refers to the therapist's attempts to communicate this understanding (Bacal, 1990). Responsiveness broadens the range of clinical inter-ventions to include mirroring, validation of an internal experience, interpretation, describing our own feelings, or working to understand and contain a difficult aspect of the patient's internal world, to simply listening. Responsiveness moves us closer toward mutuality in the process which we call intersubjectivity.

Intersubjectivity as defined by Stolorow, Atwood, and Brandchaft in the early 1980s refers to the process of reciprocal influences in which each person in the therapeutic situation influences and is influenced by the other. "Psychological phenomena cannot be understood apart from the intersubjective contexts in which they take form." It is not "the isolated mind" but rather the mutual interplay between the subjective worlds of the patient, the therapist, and/or the group where we have the most promise in the clinical experience. The concept of intersubjectivity was developed as a response to the tendency in classical analysis to assume there is an "objective reality" known by the therapist who helps the patient recognize, accept, and understand the objective reality. Stolorow advanced that the only reality is "subjective reality" (Stolorow & Atwood, 1992).

Prior to Kohut, Winnicott in 1951 makes an enormously important contribution in the shift from objectivity to subjectivity in his discussion of the use of transitional objects as intermediate between subjective and objective. Winnicott also helped us look at the role of the therapist through his conceptualizations of the "good-enough mother" and the "holding environment." As Malcolm Pines aptly states, one has to be a subject before one is an object (Klein, Bernard, & Singer, 1992).

The path to intersubjectivity was further illuminated by those who continued Margaret Mahler's work in infant research. Daniel Stem's research in the 1980s demonstrated that from neonatal and early infancy there is a mutuality, an emotional exchange between the caregiver or mother and child. Mahler spoke of the earliest phase as the autistic phase, Stern refers to the emergent phase, showing there is interaction from the earliest beginnings.

In self psychologically informed therapy, the therapist's consistent understanding of the patient's affective experience, gained through the transference, acts as a facilitating medium. It reengages the patient's natural processes of psychic growth. Sustained empathetic inquiry in the face of meeting the patient's conflicted, resistive, repetitions can provide the most growth in the clinical encounter; yet this is not easy to fulfill (Stolorow, Atwood, & Brandchaft, 1994). For the therapist, it can feel like the ground shifting or at least an insecure footing, consistently making the effort to see oneself and the world through the eyes of another. It means as therapists, we often have to contain our own anxiety, anger, or desire for how we want the patient to understand exactly what they are repeating over and over again. We have to contain the desire to interpret a situation or internal process, which first may need to be experienced and/or validated. It is true however, for treatment to be effective, old grievances, no matter how valid or legitimate, will have to be relinquished and new, more responsive or appropriate selfobjects have to be sought (Klein, Bernard, & Singer, 1992). In my experience, this does not happen on the basis of confrontation or intellectually interpreting over affect. We have all had the experience when we make what we feel is a brilliant interpretation to be responded with "so what?" or "fine, but now what do I do about it?" This probably means that the affect hasn't been engaged and that there is more beneath this interpretation. These moments fall flat on both sides.

Stolorow writes that disjunctions arising from frustration, disappointment, and experiences of misattainment are the inevitable consequences of the profoundly intersubjective nature of the analytic dialogue, the colliding of differently organized subjective galaxies (Stolorow & Atwood, 1992). Intersubjectivity challenges us as therapists to keep looking at our side of the story. Bob Winer is his book *Close Encounters* speaks of turning points in treatment (Winer, 1994). These are the places where the therapist's subjectively is engaged. This is when we have finally been able to take in or tolerate that which the patient has been struggling to tell us or show us. This is, perhaps, where we may understand feelings which have emerged in ourselves, or we are able to step away from the force field of reenacting the old history. This is where we struggle to the thirdness Ogden speaks of and are truly there for the patient. This is the moment of optimal responsiveness (Bacal, 1990), when meaning is derived by consensus, where we can both be a mirror and a window for our patients (Klein, Bernard, & Singer, 1992).

References

Bacal, H. A., & Newman, K. M. (1990). *Theories of object relations: Bridges to self psychology.* New York: Columbia University Press.

Klein, R., Bernard, H., & Singer, D. (Eds.). (1992). *Handbook of contemporary group psychotherapy.* Madison, CT: International Universities Press.

Kohut, H. (1984). *How does analysis cure?* Eds. A. Goldberg & P. Stepansky. Chicago: University of Chicago Press.

Stolorow, R. D., & Atwood, G. E. (1992). *The context of being.* Hillsdale, NJ: The Analytic Press.

Stolorow, R., Atwood, G., & Brandchaft, B. (Eds.). (1994). *The intersubjective perspective.* Northvale, NJ: Jason Aronson.

Winer, R. (1994). *Close encounters: A relational view of the therapeutic process.* Northvale, NJ: Jason Aronson.

Conclusion

Researchers, Third-Party Payers, and the Singular Group Therapist

MORRIS B. PARLOFF

Ladies and gentlemen, I am deeply honored to have been invited to participate in this, the first certificate award ceremony of the National Group Therapy Institute. I am delighted to add my sincere and enthusiastic congratulations to each of the students and to their devoted faculty.

I recognize that these sorts of occasions are intended more as moments of ritual and celebration than as platforms for the pronouncement of profundities. However, as many of your well know, I am by nature and training prone to speak profundities. I shall not now stifle that impulse lest it pop out later at an even less opportune moment.

In the past I have been able confidently to assure group therapy students that instruction would equip them not only to do good but also to do well—very well. I remain, today, as confident as ever that your group therapy training will enable you skillfully and effectively to fulfill your clinical responsibilities to your patients. However, in the context of some recent whimsical changes in the policies and practices of third-party health insurance payers, the hurdles to your own economic well being have been appreciably raised.

Third-party payers no longer find it sufficient for practitioners merely to affirm that the treatments for which they seek reimbursement meet the twin criteria of "clinical need and standard professional practice." Increasingly, psychotherapists are challenged to provide "scientific evidence" confirming that the particular treatment forms they have used are effective and appropriate. I expect at this point you may have some doubts about your readiness to fulfill that specialized task.

Your training at the school has thus far provided you with extended tours of psychodynamic theories, change processes, and treatment techniques. However, because it has not encouraged you to loiter around the dark corners of psychotherapy's "scientific" outcome literature you may not feel adequately equipped to present and interpret such evidence to *health care administrators* who now clearly lust after such data. In short, you may not feel quite ready *to go forth from here.*

But not to worry. Tonight's revelry can yet go on. Fortuitously I have come prepared to fill this lacuna in your training, and to do this well within my allotted 32 minutes. I shall equip you to respond nimbly to those who would contest the existence of persuasive evidence regarding the potency of psychotherapy in general and group psychotherapy in particular.

Specifically, I shall first review the vicissitudes of outcome research findings as reflected in the development of the field of treatment research; second, I shall compare the relative efficacy of group and individual therapy; and third, I will offer a summary and conclusions.

It will be helpful to keep in mind that at least some of the insurance administrators' hyperbolic rhetoric about their fears of suffering fiscal hemorrhages has been provoked by memories of the recent past when the growth of the entire psychotherapy enterprise appeared to be totally unrestrained.

By the 1970s the psychoanalytically oriented and client centered forms of therapy coexisted with behavior modification and behavioral forms of therapy. Then cognitive behavioral therapies emerged to form a bridge between the reinforcement theories of behavior therapy and the hermeneutic principles of psychodynamic therapy.

I shall not pursue this sort of biblical "begats" account of the advent of new forms of psychotherapy for right about here generative creativity got seriously out of hand. In 1980 Herink published a book giving full descriptions of over *250* psychotherapy approaches (Herink, 1980) and by 1986 Karasu reported that his tally had reached *450* and counting (Karasu, 1986). These compendia included many cultish psychotherapy offshoots, each competing to see which could help its patients play more imaginatively with their mental blocks.

Interventions claiming therapeutic effects, if not therapeutic intent, erupted from the confines of consultation room chairs and couches and moved expansively to the floors of hotel ballrooms.

In this context therapeutic interventions shifted from delivering measured interpretations to promoting brash confrontations. These included interaction marathons, sensitivity training, sensory awareness, and screaming of the most primal kind.

Some grudging empathy for the insurer's concerns may be gained from two observations: first, no form of psychotherapy has ever been introduced without its advocates earnestly proclaiming that it would sweep aside all the buffoonery that had preceded it, and second, no form of therapy has ever been abandoned for failure to live up to that claim. We do not dismiss therapies; we merely integrate them.

Insurance companies that had the policy of routinely reimbursing psychological treatments for indefinite periods, at about 80% of the therapists' fees, chose to interpret the field's explosive expansion as supportive of their "big bank" theory of the creation of psychotherapies. The third-party payers' favorite bumper stick remains today "Shrink costs, not heads."

I now turn to the review of research evidence regarding psychotherapy's effectiveness. I shall not use slides. I learned long ago never to turn the lights out on any of my audiences. But your comprehension of the findings will not suffer. I have every confidence that when you leave this building you will find yourselves humming the results.

Provoked by the 1950s claims of Eysenck that the effects of psychotherapy failed to exceed those of spontaneous remission (Eysenck, 1952), researchers initiated the modern era of therapy outcome research. Soon they reassuringly reported that all tested forms of psychotherapy were, indeed, effective. More specifically, patients who had completed a course of psychotherapy showed both significant improvement from their own baseline states and significantly greater benefits than did treatment-eligible patients who had not received such treatment (Luborsky, Singer, & Luborsky, 1975; Lambert & Bergin, 1994). However, the treatment effects, per se, were consistently acknowledged to be relatively small (Frank, 1973).

Clearly, something had to be done to strengthen these frail and puny findings. And researchers soon succeeded in doing that. Their breakthrough contribution did not involve, as we had hoped, the discovery of more valid knowledge regarding the basic processes and mechanisms of change leading to the development of more powerful therapeutic procedures.

Instead, what finally worked was simply using a different statistical procedure for reanalyzing the old body of psychotherapy outcome studies. This method is know as meta-analysis and is a procedure for converting outcome measurement scores into a common metric—usually stated in standard deviation terms. This enables the reviewer of outcome literature to compare and combine the findings of separate studies, but even more important, to calculate their overall *treatment effect sizes* (Smith, Glass, & Miller, 1980).

The meta-analytic procedures not only showed that psychotherapy worked but for the first time it could be documented that the magnitude of its effects was large.

Unfortunately, the law of unintended consequences asserted itself. Unbidden, the meta-analysis disclosed a far less welcome finding. While it confirmed the earlier discovery that all psychotherapies appear to work, it gratuitously also confirmed the rumor that it seemed to work equally well. This new was not at all well received by practitioners or third-party payers.

The notion that no statistically significant differences had been detected among the outcomes associated with the various psychotherapies was an affront to the clinicians' cherished "specificity hypothesis" of psychotherapy, that is, particular forms of psychological interventions were particularly effective with particular problems and patients.

The compared forms of treatment had, for the most part, been carefully derived from quite different theories and utilized quite different procedures. Their effects, therefore, *should be different*. If the no difference findings were allowed to stand, this would seriously challenge therapists who had been sustained by the conviction that their particular school or form of treatment was superior to all the other therapies on the block. Clinicians much preferred to continue their "dogma eat dogma" existences.

Of equal importance was the fact that these findings were not at all reassuring to third-party payers. The evidence failed to provide them with a hoped-for basis for *withholding* reimbursement from those forms of psychotherapy that had been tested and found to be ineffective or unsafe. Surprisingly, research had failed to identify *any* such psychotherapy. Indeed, as Luborsky had popularized, the dodo verdict prevailed: "Everyone has won and all must have prizes" (Luborsky, Singer, & Luborsky, 1975).

The question then arose, how was the apparent promiscuous success of all forms of psychotherapy to be interpreted? Two major alternative explanations were proposed: first, the "no differences" finding must be an artifact of clumsy research and therefore spurious, or second, it represents a valid finding in that all psychotherapies, wittingly or unwittingly, achieve their comparable effects not because of their claimed *unique elements* but due to some *crucial shared components* (Rosenzweig, 1936; Frank & Frank, 1991).

To minimize the opportunity for such research error, investigators then adopted more and more rigorous and vigorous "efficacy" research designs. Ultimately, they *adapted* the clinical trials method from the drug research field. The clinical trials design involves the random assignment of patients manifesting a single, well-defined disorder to manualized treatments or control groups for comparable periods. Targeted outcome goals and measures are selected in advance and are administered at predetermined intervals pre-, during, and post-treatment. A number of such psychotherapy clinical trials studies have been successfully conducted over the past 20 years (e.g., Sloane, Staples, Cristol, Yorkston, & Whipple, 1975; NIMH collaborative depression study, e.g., Elkin, Parloff, Hadley, & Autry, 1985; Elkin et al., 1989; Elkin, Shea, Gibbons, & Shaw, 1996; the first Sheffield psychotherapy project, e.g., Shapiro & Firth, 1987; the second Sheffield psychotherapy project, e.g., Shapiro et al., 1990, and Startup & Shapiro, 1992).

In 1995 a task force of the American Psychological Association's Division of Clinical Psychology (Div. XII) reviewed the body of rigorously controlled studies of this kind (Task Force on Promotion and Dissemination). The task force's initial aim was to provide a list of "empirically validated treatments" to psychologists, the public, and third-party payers. By 1996, in response to the unhappy reactions of some segments of Division XII, five major revisions of the goals and procedures were made in the updated report (Chambless et al., 1996):

1. The specific aim of informing third-party payers of what therapies had been empirically supported was deleted.

2. While the term "empirically validated" was retained, its interpretation was modified to be consistent with the notion that validation had not, in fact, been accomplished but would remain a continuing process. It is now planned that annual reports will be published to present amended listings of findings that "support" validation.

3. The report would no longer to be represented as an office policy statement of Division XII but would simply list the names of its authors.

4. All empirically supported therapies were to be listed along with the names of the problems effectively treated by each.

5. Some of the criteria by which treatments were classified as either empirically validated or probably efficacious were modified.

As many of you know, the results clearly supported the specificity hypothesis. Results were classified under two headings: "Well-Established Treatments" and "Probably Efficacious Treatments," as follows.

Well-Established Treatments

The well-established treatments list includes the names of psychological approaches found, by well-designed research (or by a cumulative series of well-designed case studies), to be especially suited for the treatment of specific problems and disorders. I have opened the envelope and the winners in this category are as follows:

- *Interpersonal therapy* is listed in 1995 as an effective treatment for only two problems—bulimia and depression. More specifically, it is the Klerman and Weissman version of *interpersonal therapy* that was found to be an effective treatment for major depressive disorder.
- *Cognitive behavior therapy* is also listed an effective with depression. In addition, it is described as effective with a wide range of problems—for example, panic disorders (with and without agoraphobia), generalized anxiety disorder, irritable bowel syndrome, opiate dependence, and chronic pain. In addition, the *group therapy version of cognitive behavioral therapy* is depicted as effective for social phobia.
- *Behavior therapy* is listed as a broad spectrum treatment for problems such as headaches, childhood enuresis, and adult sexual dysfunctions. Behavioral marital therapy is recorded as effective for "marital discord."
- *Exposure treatment* is named as effective with agoraphobia, obsessive-compulsive disorder, and social phobia.

- And finally, *response prevention* is mentioned as useful in the treatment of obsessive-compulsive disorder.

Probably Efficacious Treatments

- In 1995 *brief dynamic therapy* was included without specifying the problems or disorders it usefully treated. The 1996 report corrects this oversight.
- *Dynamic therapy* may be an effective treatment both for opiate dependence and depression among the aged.
- *Insight-oriented* treatment continues in 1996 to be listed as probably efficacious in the area of marital problems. Similarly, *"emotionally focused" couples therapy* is also listed as appropriate for ameliorating marital discord.
- *Cognitive therapy* is described as probably useful with opiate disorders, depression in geriatric patients, and *group cognitive-behavior therapy* is recorded as a likely treatment for bulimia.
- *Applied relaxation* may be useful for panic disorder and generalized anxiety.
- *Behavior therapy* for encopresis had initially been listed in 1995 as an "empirically validated" treatment. However, in the 1996 report it is downgraded to the category of "probably" efficacious treatments. Despite the recent spate of reports in the media regarding the high recidivism rate among sex offenders, *behavior modification* continues to be cited in the 1996 report as probably effective with such individuals.
- *Dialectical behavior therapy*, as developed by Marsha Linehan (1993), continues to be the only treatment recognized as probably useful in the treatment of borderline personality disorder.
- *Group exposure, response prevention,* and *relapse prevention* are reported as probably effective techniques for obsessive-compulsive disorder.
- *Stress inoculation training* and *exposure treatment* are both cited as treatments for PTSD.

Thus, the closest approximation to any psychodynamic form of therapy found in the 1995 and 1996 lists of the *well-established treatment* category is *interpersonal therapy*. However, thus far it has been demonstrated to be effective only with bulimia and depression. These findings, while welcome, provide but small comfort to those clinicians who believe that the unique advantages of dynamic therapy have not been acknowledged.

Further, dynamically oriented therapists may not be much reassured to learn that under the category of *probably efficacious treatments*, *brief dynamic therapy* is listed only for depression among the aged and the general care of opiate dependence, while *insight-oriented* treatment per se is catalogued only as a probably useful form of marital therapy.

Thus, by the criteria of rigorous efficacy research the psychodynamic therapies have thus far, earned only a tenuous position on either the *well-established treatments* or *probably efficacious treatments* lists.

There is, of course, an obvious caution to be observed in interpreting these findings. The mere absence of a form of psychotherapy or a problem category from the above two slates is not to be interpreted as evidence that they have been tested and found to be wanting. It is far more likely that they have not been tested. Most of the rigorous studies have been performed on the behavioral and cognitive therapies rather than the psychodynamic. *And the dynamic therapists, if the truth be known, would have it no other way.*

The psychotherapy researchers' single-minded devotion to the *efficacy* or randomized clinical trials (RCT) model appears recently to have reached its apogee. Among the indicators of such a shift, the most important way may be the growing consensus that while findings derived from the RCT's sanitized laboratory conditions are necessary for the task of inferring "cause-effect" relationships between specified interventions and specified changes, the findings from RCT cannot be easily generalized to the less orderly world of clinical practice. For this pragmatic task, adaptations of the *effectiveness* research model may be more useful.

In the lead article of the December 1995 issue of *American Psychologist* (Seligman, 1995) the distinctions between efficacy and effectiveness research were emphasized and a surprisingly enthusiastic endorsement was given of the more casual effectiveness research model. Specifically, what was lauded was a large-scale *naturalistic psychotherapy outcome survey* conducted by *Consumer Reports* and published in November 1995 ("Mental Health," 1995).

That survey was based on reports from 2900 patients regarding the effectiveness of their own therapy with professional psychotherapists. The treatment forms were nonstandardized, were of variable duration, and were provided to patients who may have been multiply-disordered. Five of its major findings are these.

1. Respondents generally reported that they had gotten "a lot better" during treatment independent of whether their therapist had been a psychiatrist, social worker, or psychologist.

2. No specific modality of psychotherapy did any better than any other for any problems treated.

3. *Long-term therapy produced more improvement than short-term therapy.* This was described as a very robust finding. (It certainly supports the long-held view of dynamically oriented therapists.)

4. Patients who *actively sought treatment and participated in the selection of their therapists did better in treatment than patients who passively accepted therapist assignment.*

5. Respondents whose choice of therapists or duration of care was limited by their insurance carriers did worse!!

These are very provocative findings. But in this context let's bash on to the information you have been eagerly awaiting, namely, the comparative efficacy of group and individual therapy.

What I shall report is an abridgment of my testimony on behalf of the American Group Psychotherapy Association before two congressional committees dealing with health care reimbursement legislation (Subcommittee on Health, 1993; Subcommittee on Health and the Environment, 1993).

My review was based on a body of over 280 comparisons of the relative effectiveness of group and individual therapy in the treatment of outpatient *adults*. The salient findings are these:

- Both group and individual psychotherapy are clinically very effective.
- Most of the comparisons of the effects of group and individual therapy did not reveal any statistically significant differences, but when such differences were found they tended to favor group therapy.
- From the point of view of clinicians and clinic administrators there is now ample evidence to justify giving priority to the expanded use of group psychotherapy.
- In terms of demonstrated effectiveness, efficiency, and cost-effectiveness to patients, therapists, and sponsoring agencies group psychotherapy has much to commend it to health care administrators.

In summary, you can tell third-party payers that when psychotherapy outcome findings are collated among and between efficacy and effectiveness research studies the following eight-point consensus is achieved:

1. Patients received clinically and statistically significant benefit from all tested forms of psychotherapy including group therapy.

2. Efficacy studies reveal that some behavioral and cognitive therapies appear to be especially useful in the treatment of patients manifesting designated symptoms and symptom patterns.

3. Effectiveness studies of psychotherapy have recently provided dramatic support for the claimed benefits of psychotherapy as generally practiced.

4. No consistent differences in treatment benefits have been found among patients treated by members of the three major psychotherapy professions.

5. A strong positive association was found between the amount of patient-benefit and the patients' active participation in the selection of their therapist.

6. Long-term psychotherapy is more effective in producing and maintaining symptom relief, enhancing general functioning and improving quality of life than is short-term therapy.

7. Patients whose length of therapy or choice of therapist was limited by third-party payers did not do nearly as well. Thus, long-term therapy may ultimately be cost-effective, especially with specific types of problems.

8. The findings derived from the comparison of group and individual therapy also revealed that group therapy was not only effective but inherently cost effective.

Ladies and gentlemen, in acknowledgment of the solemn aspect of this festive occasion I wish to offer two final comments:

The first takes the form of a time-honored benediction and is especially appropriate for all who would distinguish between professional training and vocational indoctrination. It was first passed on to me by my late dear friend, the Reverend John Porter. John said, "May you *never* cease your quest after the truth, and may you *always* be spared the company of those who are absolutely convinced they have found it."

And second, you will recall that at the beginning of this talk I suggested that you might not be quite ready to go. *Now*, you are ready.

References

Chambless, D., Sanderson, W., Shoham, V., Johnson, S., Pope, K., Crits-Christoph, P., Baker, M., Johnson, B., Woody, S., Sue, S., Beutler, L., Williams, D., & McCurry, S. (1996). An update on empirically validated therapies. *The Clinical Psychologist, 49*, 5–18.

Elkin, I., Parloff, M., Hadley, S., & Autry, J. (1985). NIMH Treatment of Depression Collaborative Research Program: Background and research plan. *Archives of General Psychiatry, 42*, 305–316.

Elkin, I., Shea, T., Gibbons, R., & Shaw, B. (1996). Science is not a trial (but it can sometimes be a tribulation). *Journal of Consulting and Clinical Psychology, 64*, 92–103.

Elkin, I., Shea, T., Imber, S., Sotsky, S., Collins, J., Glass, D., Pilkonis, P., Leber, W., Docherty, J., Fiester, S., & Parloff, M. (1989). National Institute of Mental Health treatment of Depression Collaborative Research Program: General effectiveness of treatments. *Archives of General Psychiatry, 46*, 971–982.

Eysenck, H. J. (1952). The effects of psychotherapy: An evaluation. *Journal of Consulting Psychology, 16*, 319–324.

Frank, J. D. (1973). *Persuasion and healing* (2nd ed.). Baltimore: Johns Hopkins University Press.

Frank, J. D., & Frank, J. B. (1991). *Persuasion and healing.* Baltimore: Johns Hopkins University Press.

Herink, R. (Ed.). (1980). *The psychotherapy handbook.* New York: New American Library.

Karasu, T. B. (1986). The psychotherapies: Benefits and limitations. *American Journal of Psychotherapy, 40*, 324–342.

Lambert, M. J., & Bergin, A. E. (1994). The effectiveness of psychotherapy. In A. E. Bergin & S. L. Garfield (Eds.), *Handbook of psychotherapy and behavior change* (4th ed., pp. 143–189). New York: Wiley.

Linehan, M. (1993). *Cognitive-behavioral treatment of borderline personality disorder.* New York: Guilford Press.

Luborsky, L., Singer, H., & Luborsky, I. (1975). Comparative studies of psychotherapies. *Archives of General Psychiatry, 32*, 995–1008.

Mental health: Does therapy help? (1995, November). *Consumer Reports,* 734–739.

Rosenzweig, S. (1936). Some implicit common factors in diverse methods of psychotherapy. *American Journal of Orthopsychiatry, 6*, 412–415.

Seligman, M. (1995). The effectiveness of psychotherapy: The *Consumer Reports* study. *American Psychologist, 50*, 965–974.

Shapiro, D., Barkham, M., Hardy, G., Morrison, L., Reynolds, S., Startup, M., & Harper, H. (1990). University of Sheffield Psychotherapy Research Program: Medical Research Council/Economic and Social Research Council Social and Applied Psychology Unit. In L. E. Beutler & M. Crago (Eds.), *Psychotherapy research programs* (pp. 234–242). Washington, DC: American Psychological Association.

Shapiro, D., & Firth, J. (1987). Prescriptive vs. exploratory psychotherapy: Outcomes of the Sheffield Psychotherapy Project. *British Journal of Psychiatry, 151*, 790–799.

Sloane, R., Staples, F., Cristol, A., Yorkston, N., & Whipple, K. (1975). *Psychotherapy versus behavior therapy.* Cambridge, MA: Harvard University Press.

Smith, M., Glass, G., & Miller, T. (1980). *The benefits of psychotherapy.* Baltimore: Johns Hopkins University Press.

Startup, M., & Shapiro, D. (1992). *Therapist treatment fidelity in prescriptive vs. exploratory psychotherapy* (SAPU Memo 1263). Sheffield: University of Sheffield.

Subcommittee on Health—House Ways and Means Committee, March 30, 1993.

Subcommittee on Health and the Environment—House Energy and Commerce Committee, Dec. 6, 1993.

Task Force on Promotion and Dissemination of Psychological Procedures Division of Clinical Psychology, American Psychological Association. Training in and dissemination of empirically-validated psychological treatment: Report and recommendations. *The Clinical Psychologist, 50*, 3–23.

Index

www.ingramcontent.com/pod-product-compliance
Ingram Content Group UK Ltd.
Pitfield, Milton Keynes, MK11 3LW, UK
UKHW020433010325
455677UK00029B/1132